The ... of acu... infe... ...en

Pract...
outpa...

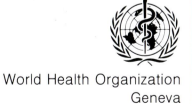

World Health Organization
Geneva

3/11/99
M

WHO Library Cataloguing in Publication Data

The management of acute respiratory infections in children :
    practical guidelines for outpatient care.

    1.Respiratory tract infections — in infancy & childhood 2.Patient care planning 3.Child care
    4.Guidelines

    ISBN 92 4 154477 5   (NLM Classification: WS 280)

The designations employed and the presentation of the material in this publication do not imply the expression of any opinion whatsoever on the part of the Secretariat of the World Health Organization concerning the legal status of any country, city or area or of its authorities, or concerning the delimitation of its frontiers or boundaries.

The mention of specific companies or of certain manufacturers' products does not imply that they are endorsed or recommended by the World Health Organization in preference to others of a similar nature that are not mentioned. Errors and omissions excepted, the names of proprietary products are distinguished by initial capital letters.

Typeset in India
Printed in France
94/9926 – Macmillan/Sadag – 8500

Contents

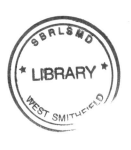

Foreword

This book is intended for supervisors or other health staff working in first-level health facilities who are responsible for managing children with acute respiratory infections (ARI). The guidelines form the technical basis of the module entitled "Supervisory Skills: Management of the Young Child with an Acute Respiratory Infection", a training course of the World Health Organization.[1] Staff from referral facilities or facilities with the capability to give inpatient care to severely ill children with acute respiratory infections should refer to the document *Acute respiratory infections in children: case management in small hospitals in developing countries. A manual for doctors and other senior health workers*.[1]

The three steps to correct management of a child with a respiratory infection are: assess the child, classify the illness, and treat. Two fold-out charts are provided at the back of the book which summarize this approach to case management for acute respiratory infections. These are: "Management of the Child with Cough or Difficult Breathing" and "Management of the Child with an Ear Problem or Sore Throat". The three steps, and the sections of the management charts that describe them, are explained in this book.

- The chapter on assessment describes how to collect the information needed about signs of respiratory problems.
- The chapters on classifying the illness explain how to use the signs to classify the illness and identify the appropriate treatment.
- The chapters on treatment describe how to: give an antibiotic, advise the mother on how to give home care, treat fever, treat wheezing, and wick dry a draining ear.

At the end of each chapter, there is a list of the essential skills and knowledge required by health workers for the management of acute respiratory infections. A summary of the essential skills and knowledge is given in Annex 1. At the end of the book, there is a section that defines the technical words used in this book. Refer to that section whenever you read an unfamiliar term.

---

[1] The documents mentioned in this book should be available from the national ARI programme in your country. If you have any difficulty, however, the documents may be obtained from the Division of Diarrhoeal and Acute Respiratory Disease Control (CDR), World Health Organization, 1211 Geneva 27, Switzerland.

CHAPTER 1
Introduction

Understanding the problem

Most children have about 4–6 acute respiratory infections each year. Children with respiratory infections account for a large proportion of patients seen by health workers in health centres. These infections tend to be even more frequent in urban communities than in rural areas.

Respiratory infections are infections in any area of the respiratory tract, including the nose, middle ear, throat (pharynx), voice box (larynx), windpipe (trachea), air passages (bronchi or bronchioles), and lungs (see Fig. 1).

Many areas of the respiratory tract can be involved, and there can be a wide variety of signs and symptoms of infection. These include:

— cough;
— difficult breathing;
— sore throat;
— runny nose;
— ear problems.

Fever is also common in acute respiratory infections. Fortunately, most children with these respiratory symptoms have only a mild infection, such as a cold or bronchitis. They may cough because nasal discharge from a cold drips down the back of the throat, or because they have a viral infection of the bronchi (bronchitis). They are not seriously ill and can be treated at home by their families without antibiotics.

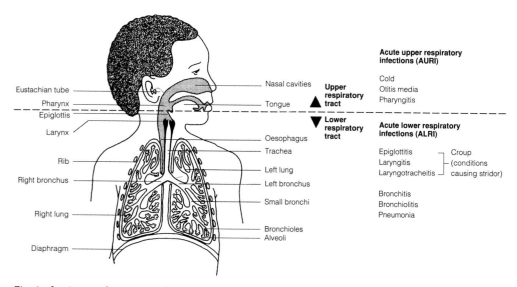

Fig. 1. **Acute respiratory syndromes: clinical syndromes**

However, a few children have an acute infection of the lungs (pneumonia). If they are not treated with an antibiotic, these children may die, either from a lack of oxygen, or from a bacterial infection of the bloodstream (called sepsis or septicaemia). About one-quarter of all children less than 5 years of age who die in developing countries do so because of pneumonia. Pneumonia and diarrhoea are the two most common causes of death in children. Many of the deaths from pneumonia occur in young infants less than 2 months of age.[1]

Therefore, treating children who have pneumonia can greatly reduce deaths in children. In order to treat these children, the health worker must be able to carry out the difficult task of identifying the few, very sick children among the many children with respiratory infections that are not serious.

Selecting the appropriate case management chart

The two fold-out case management charts included at the back of this book summarize the management steps for different illnesses. Therefore, one of the first steps in managing a child with an acute respiratory infection is to determine which of the two charts to use. To do this:

1. Welcome the mother and ask her to sit with the child.

2. Ask her why she has come.

3. If the mother's response does not include cough or difficult breathing, ask her if the child has a cough or has difficult breathing.

   - It is important to ask the mother this question because mothers will often simply say that their child has a cold or a runny nose, and not specify that the child also has a cough or difficult breathing.
   - "Difficult breathing" refers to any unusual pattern of breathing in a child. Mothers may describe it in different ways. For example, they might use the terms "noisy", "fast", or "interrupted".
   - A young infant may have pneumonia or another severe disease without coughing, so health workers should be particularly careful when listening to mothers describe symptoms of a young infant to determine whether there is a history of difficult breathing.

4. If the mother's response still does not include cough or difficult breathing, look to see if the child is coughing or has difficult breathing.

5. Then, select the appropriate case management chart:

   - If the mother's response or your observation includes cough or difficult breathing, use the chart, "Management of the child with cough or difficult breathing".
   - If the child has an ear problem or a sore throat (without a cough or difficult breathing), use the chart, "Management of the child with an ear problem or sore throat".

---

[1] Throughout this book, the term "young infant" is used to refer to an infant less than 2 months of age.

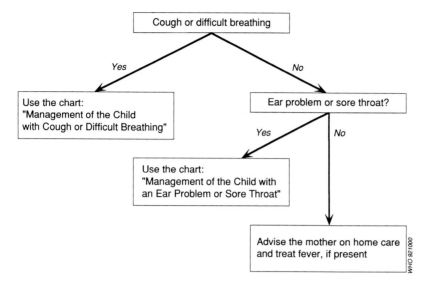

Fig. 2. **Decision tree for selecting the appropriate case management chart**

- If the child has a cough or difficult breathing, and an ear problem or sore throat, first use the chart, "Management of the child with cough or difficult breathing".
- If the child has a runny nose or cold (without a cough, difficult breathing, an ear problem or a sore throat), the child needs home care only. Advise the mother how to give home care and treat any fever, if present.

Fig. 2 summarizes how to select the appropriate case management chart for assessing, classifying and treating acute respiratory infections.

Essential skills and knowledge

By the end of this chapter, you should be able to select the appropriate case management chart for assessing, classifying and treating acute respiratory infections:

- For a child with a cough or difficult breathing, use the chart, "Management of the Child with Cough or Difficult Breathing".
- For a child with only an ear problem or sore throat, use the chart, "Management of the Child with an Ear Problem or Sore Throat".

PART 1

Management of the child with cough or difficult breathing

CHAPTER 2
Assessing a child who has cough or difficult breathing

"Assessing" a child means obtaining information about the child's illness by asking the mother questions, and looking at and listening to the child. This chapter describes what information to obtain about the child, and how to obtain it.

A child with a cough or difficult breathing could have pneumonia, which is a serious disease that can result in death. However, a cough or difficult breathing can also be caused by a common cold, a blocked nose, a dusty environment, whooping cough (pertussis), tuberculosis, measles, croup or wheezing disorders. (Annex 2 describes how to recognize and manage acute respiratory infections caused by the vaccine-preventable diseases, measles, pertussis and diphtheria.) Careful assessment of a child can help to prevent deaths from pneumonia and other severe diseases.

The steps for assessing a child are presented here and given on the fold-out chart "Management of the Child with Cough or Difficult Breathing" under the title "Assess". You should first ask the mother certain questions about the child's health. You should then look at and listen to the child for signs of difficult breathing and general signs of the child's condition.[1]

Below is the section of the chart that lists the points to cover during the assessment.

ASK:

- How old is the child?
- Is the child coughing? For how long?
- Age 2 months up to 5 years: Is the child able to drink?
  Age less than 2 months: Has the young infant stopped feeding well?
- Has the child had fever? For how long?
- Has the child had convulsions?

LOOK, LISTEN:

(Child must be calm)

- Count the breaths in one minute.
- Look for chest indrawing.
- Look and listen for stridor.
- Look and listen for wheeze. Is it recurrent?

- See if the child is abnormally sleepy, or difficult to wake.
- Feel for fever, or low body temperature (or measure temperature).
- Look for severe malnutrition.

---

[1] If a child is obviously very sick and in need of care that you cannot provide, the child should be referred to a hospital immediately without assessment. The assessment process described in this book considers only the steps to follow to identify respiratory infections or other related illnesses.

In many clinics, screening for immunization status is routinely done for all young children. For additional information on immunization screening, see the training module entitled "Plan to provide immunization services" in "EPI training for mid-level managers", available through your national immunization programme.

It is important to keep the child as calm as possible because a child who is crying and upset may exhibit signs that can be confused with signs of illness. Before beginning the assessment, ask the mother:

- *Not* to wake up the child, if the child is asleep.
- *Not* to undress or disturb the child.

Then start the assessment. As you cover each point, record your findings on a piece of paper so that you can remember them.

What to ask the mother

Ask the mother (or caregiver) the following questions:

- **How old is the child?**

- **Is the child coughing? For how long?**

- **Age 2 months up to 5 years: is the child able to drink?**
  The child should only be regarded as "not able to drink" if he or she is not able to drink *at all*. This includes the child who is too weak to drink when offered fluids, is not able to suck or swallow, or who repeatedly vomits and keeps nothing down.

  Children who are breast-fed may have difficulty sucking when their noses are blocked. However, if they are not severely ill, they can still breast-feed if their noses are cleared.

- **Age less than 2 months: has the young infant stopped feeding well?**
  This question is similar to the one listed above. The difference between the two questions, however, is that the sign in the older child is "not able to drink *at all*". In the young infant, the sign is taking *less than half* of the usual amount of breast milk or formula. Mothers can estimate changes in the amount of milk taken from the length of time the child sucks.

- **Has the child had fever? For how long?**

- **Has the child had convulsions?**
  Ask the mother if the child has had convulsions during the current illness.

What to look at and listen for

This section describes how to look at and listen to a child to find out whether the child has signs of difficult breathing such as chest indrawing, fast breathing, stridor or wheeze.

It is especially important to look at and listen to the child's breathing only when the child is quiet and calm. It is not possible to count the breathing rate accurately or assess other signs of difficult breathing in a child who is frightened, crying or angry. To calm the child, give the child something to play with, ask the mother to breast-feed the child, or suggest they wait in another room until the child calms down.

- **Count the breaths in one minute.**

  Look for breathing movement anywhere on the child's chest or abdomen. If you are not able to see this movement easily, ask the mother to lift the child's shirt. If the child starts to cry or becomes upset, ask the mother to calm the child again before counting.

  As children get older, their breathing rate slows down. Therefore, the cut-off you will use to determine if a child has fast breathing will depend on the age of the child (see below).

If the child is:	Then he or she has fast breathing if you count:
Aged less than 2 months	60 breaths per minute or more
Aged 2 months up to 12 months[a]	50 breaths per minute or more
Aged 12 months up to 5 years[b]	40 breaths per minute or more

[a] "Up to 12 months" means up to and including the day before the child's first birthday.
[b] "Up to 5 years" means including the day before the child's fifth birthday. Therefore, a child who is exactly 12 months old would have fast breathing if he or she breathed 40 or more times per minute.

Three useful methods for counting a child's breaths are:[1]

1. Use a sounding timer that sounds after one minute (60 seconds). Count the child's breaths for one minute.

2. Use a watch with a second hand or a digital watch. Ask another person to tell you when 60 seconds have passed so that you can watch the child's chest. If you cannot find anyone to help you, put the watch where you can glance at the second hand while looking at the child's chest to count the breaths.

3. Use a watch with a second hand or a digital watch. Count to the breathing rate cut-off (60, 50 or 40, according to the age of the child), then look back at the watch to see if this took more than one minute.

Repeat the count of a child aged 2 months up to 5 years if you are unsure of the count (e.g. if the child was moving and it was difficult to watch the chest).

However, repeat the count of a young infant *every* time you count 60 breaths per minute or more. This is important because the breathing rate of young infants is often erratic. Young infants will occasionally stop breathing for a few seconds, and then breathe very rapidly for a short period. This is why it is also important to count the young infant's breathing for a full 60 seconds. Determine if a young infant has fast breathing in this way:

- If you count less than 60 breaths per minute, the young infant does not have fast breathing.

---

[1] These methods can also be used with a half-minute count for children aged 2 months up to 5 years. For children aged 2 months up to 12 months, fast breathing is 25 breaths or more per half minute; for children aged 12 months up to 5 years, fast breathing is 20 breaths or more per half minute. However, for young infants, it is important to count for a full minute because their breathing rate is often irregular.

- If you count a rate of 60 breaths or more, wait for a few minutes and repeat the count:
  - if the second count is also 60 or more breaths per minute, the young infant has fast breathing.
  - if the second count is less than 60 breaths per minute, the young infant does not have fast breathing.

If you have not already done so, ask the mother to lift the child's shirt before you look and listen for chest indrawing, stridor and wheeze. Before looking for these signs, make sure you know when the child is breathing in and when the child is breathing out.

- **Look for chest indrawing.**

  Look for chest indrawing when the child breathes in. The child has chest indrawing if *the lower chest wall goes in when the child breathes in*. Chest indrawing occurs when the effort required to breathe in is much greater than normal. In normal breathing, when the child breathes in, the whole chest wall (upper and lower) and the abdomen move out (Fig. 3a). With chest indrawing, when the child breathes in, the lower chest wall moves in, while the upper chest wall and abdomen move out (Fig. 3b). If only the soft tissue between the ribs or above the clavicle goes in when the child breathes in (intercostal retraction), this is not chest indrawing.[1]

(a) A child breathing in *without* chest indrawing

(b) A child breathing in *with* chest indrawing

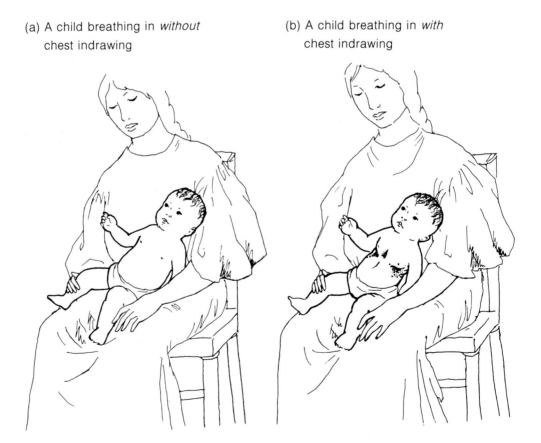

Fig. 3. **Identifying chest indrawing**

---

[1] Chest indrawing as defined here is the same as "subcostal indrawing" or "subcostal retraction".

Be especially careful when looking for chest indrawing in young infants. Mild chest indrawing is normal in young infants because their chest wall bones are soft. However, severe chest indrawing (very deep and easy to see) is a sign of pneumonia.

If you are not certain whether the child has chest indrawing, reposition the child and look again. If the child's body is bent at the waist, it is hard to judge the movement of the lower chest wall. The child should be lying flat in the mother's lap. If chest indrawing is not visible when the child is in this position, assume that the child does not have this sign.

Chest indrawing is only significant if it is present all the time and clearly visible. If you see it only when the child is upset or trying to feed, but not when the child is resting peacefully, do not count this as chest indrawing.

- **Look and listen for stridor.**

  Look to see when the child is breathing in. A child with stridor makes a harsh noise when breathing in. Listen for stridor by holding your ear near the child's mouth, since the noise may be difficult to hear. Stridor occurs when there is a narrowing of the larynx, trachea or epiglottis which interferes with air entering the lungs. These conditions are often called croup.

  Sometimes you will hear a wet noise if the child's nose is blocked. Clear the nose and listen again. Often, a child who is not very ill will have stridor only when he or she is crying or upset, so be sure to look and listen for stridor when the child is calm.

- **Look and listen for wheeze. Is it recurrent?**

  Look to see when the child is breathing out. A child with wheezing makes a soft whistling noise or shows signs that breathing out is difficult. Listen for wheeze by holding your ear near the child's mouth, since the noise may be difficult to hear. Wheezing is caused by a narrowing of the air passages in the lungs. The breathing-out phase takes longer than normal and requires effort.

  Sometimes so little air moves that there is no noise. Look to see if the breathing-out phase requires effort, and is longer than normal.

  If the child is wheezing, ask the mother if her child has had a previous episode of wheezing within the past year. If so, the child should be classified as having recurrent wheeze.

It is also important to look at and listen to the child for other signs of the child's general condition. These signs are listed below and can be assessed even when the child is not calm.

- **See if the child is abnormally sleepy or difficult to wake.**

  An abnormally sleepy child is drowsy most of the time when he or she should be awake and alert, and often will not look at the mother or watch your face when you talk. The child may stare blankly and may not appear to see.

  Ask the mother if the child has seemed unusually sleepy or difficult to wake. Look to see if the child wakens when the mother talks or when you clap your hands. A child who is difficult to wake may continue to sleep even with the mother's voice or a loud clap. Even very young babies, who sleep a lot, should waken naturally with these disturbances, or when their mother begins to undress them.

- **Feel for fever or low body temperature (or measure temperature).**

Measure the child's temperature, if possible. A temperature of 38 °C[1] or above is regarded as fever. Below 35.5 °C[2] is an abnormally low body temperature, called hypothermia.[3]

If you do not have a thermometer, feel the child's body to see if it is hot or too cold. Sometimes the hands and feet may feel cold in a child who is not adequately wrapped. However, cold calves and armpits indicate that the child is hypothermic (too cold).

- **Check for severe malnutrition.**

Check for severe malnutrition by looking at the child.[4] Look for:

- Severe marasmus, which is characterized by severe muscle wasting and a lack of subcutaneous fat, so that the child looks like skin and bones.
- Kwashiorkor, which is characterized by a generalized swelling of the body (oedema), dry, flaking skin, and thin, weak hair (Fig. 4).

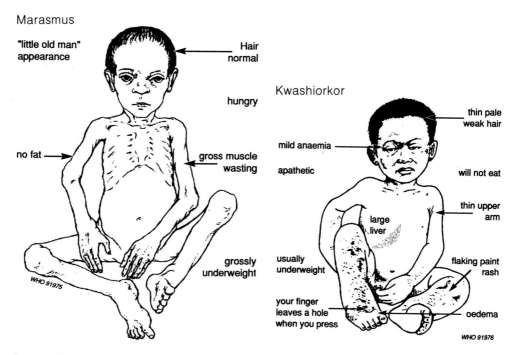

Fig. 4. **Clinical features of marasmus and kwashiorkor**

---

[1] The Fahrenheit equivalent for 38 °C is 100.4 °F.

[2] The Fahrenheit equivalent for 35.5 °C is 96 °F. These thresholds are based on rectal temperature. The thresholds for axillary temperature readings are approximately 0.5 °C lower.

[3] Ensure that the thermometer is capable of reading below 36 °C.

[4] Other methods can be used to determine if a child is severely malnourished, such as measuring weight and height, or the circumference of the arm. Follow the policy of your national maternal and child health programme.

Essential skills and knowledge

By the end of this chapter, you should be able to assess a child (ask, look and listen) for danger signs of very severe disease and pneumonia, and check for other signs of the child's general condition.

CHAPTER 3
Classifying the illness of the child aged 2 months up to 5 years

In the previous chapter you learned how to assess a child who has a cough or difficult breathing. In this chapter you will learn how to interpret the signs for a child aged 2 months up to 5 years,[1] classify the child's illness, and identify the appropriate treatment for that illness.

"Classifying the illness" means making decisions about the type and severity of disease. This is done by answering questions about the signs seen during the assessment. Each child should be put into one of four classifications:

- Very severe disease.
- Severe pneumonia.
- Pneumonia (not severe).
- No pneumonia: cough or cold.

Each disease classification has a corresponding treatment plan which should be followed after the child's illness has been classified. There are three general treatment plans, although there will be minor variations depending on the child's age, whether the child has fever or is wheezing, and whether referral is feasible.

Refer to the fold-out case management chart and find the title, "Classify the illness". Note that the boxes in this section are either red, yellow or green. Each colour refers to one of the three general treatment plans.

- Red means, "refer urgently to hospital".
- Yellow means, "give an antibiotic plus home care".
- Green means, "give home care".

The colour of the boxes will help to determine the severity of the illness and the appropriate treatment plan quickly.

The age of the child is the first piece of information used from the assessment. This is important because a different section of the chart is appropriate when a child aged 2 months up to 5 years is classified than when a young infant is classified. Under the title, "Classify the illness" on the fold-out case management chart, find the subheading, "The child age 2 months up to 5 years".

Use the boxes below this subheading to manage a child who is 2 months up to 5 years of age. These boxes are reproduced below.

---

[1] Young infants die more often of pneumonia, and are therefore managed somewhat differently from older children. This chapter describes how to classify the illness of a child aged 2 months up to 5 years (i.e. 2–59 months of age). The next chapter describes how to classify the illness of young infants (i.e. aged less than 2 months).

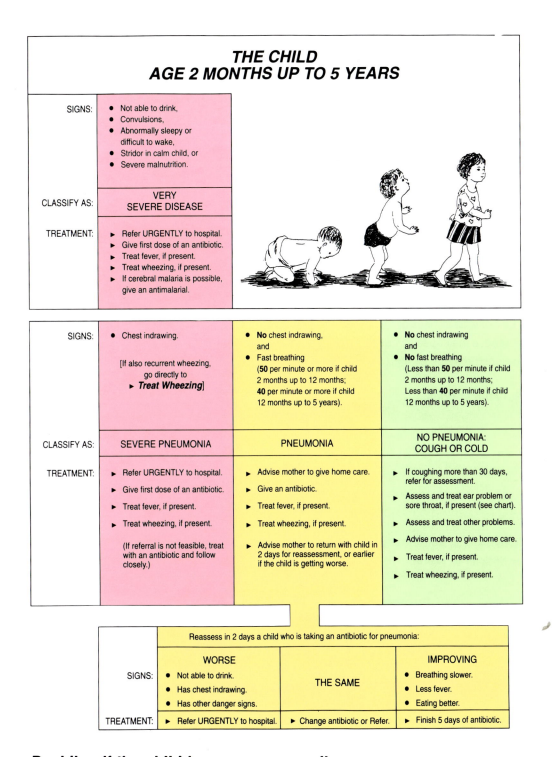

THE CHILD
AGE 2 MONTHS UP TO 5 YEARS

SIGNS:	• Not able to drink, • Convulsions, • Abnormally sleepy or difficult to wake, • Stridor in calm child, or • Severe malnutrition.		
CLASSIFY AS:	**VERY SEVERE DISEASE**		
TREATMENT:	▸ Refer URGENTLY to hospital. ▸ Give first dose of an antibiotic. ▸ Treat fever, if present. ▸ Treat wheezing, if present. ▸ If cerebral malaria is possible, give an antimalarial.		

SIGNS:	• Chest indrawing. [If also recurrent wheezing, go directly to ▸ *Treat Wheezing*]	• **No** chest indrawing, and • **Fast** breathing (**50** per minute or more if child 2 months up to 12 months; **40** per minute or more if child 12 months up to 5 years).	• **No** chest indrawing and • **No** fast breathing (Less than **50** per minute if child 2 months up to 12 months; Less than **40** per minute if child 12 months up to 5 years).
CLASSIFY AS:	**SEVERE PNEUMONIA**	**PNEUMONIA**	**NO PNEUMONIA: COUGH OR COLD**
TREATMENT:	▸ Refer URGENTLY to hospital. ▸ Give first dose of an antibiotic. ▸ Treat fever, if present. ▸ Treat wheezing, if present. (If referral is not feasible, treat with an antibiotic and follow closely.)	▸ Advise mother to give home care. ▸ Give an antibiotic. ▸ Treat fever, if present. ▸ Treat wheezing, if present. ▸ Advise mother to return with child in 2 days for reassessment, or earlier if the child is getting worse.	▸ If coughing more than 30 days, refer for assessment. ▸ Assess and treat ear problem or sore throat, if present (see chart). ▸ Assess and treat other problems. ▸ Advise mother to give home care. ▸ Treat fever, if present. ▸ Treat wheezing, if present.

	Reassess in 2 days a child who is taking an antibiotic for pneumonia:		
SIGNS:	**WORSE** • Not able to drink. • Has chest indrawing. • Has other danger signs.	**THE SAME**	**IMPROVING** • Breathing slower. • Less fever. • Eating better.
TREATMENT:	▸ Refer URGENTLY to hospital.	▸ Change antibiotic or Refer.	▸ Finish 5 days of antibiotic.

Deciding if the child has very severe disease

As stated earlier, there are four classifications of disease for a child aged 2 months up to 5 years: very severe disease, severe pneumonia, pneumonia (not severe), and no pneumonia: cough or cold. To classify the child's illness, you should follow the steps presented in this section of the book. The first step is to decide if the child should be classified as having very severe disease.

You can tell if a child has very severe disease by using the information from the assessment to decide if the child has a "danger sign". *You should ask this question about every child with a cough or difficult breathing.*

15

- **Does the child have danger signs?**

A child who has:
any danger sign
is classified as having very severe disease

Danger signs for the child aged 2 months up to 5 years of age are:

— not able to drink;
— convulsions;
— abnormally sleepy or difficult to wake;
— stridor when calm;
— severe malnutrition.

The possible causes of these signs are many; however, health workers are not required to diagnose their specific cause. They need only to recognize the danger signs and know that the child may be at high risk of dying.

Not able to drink:

A child who is not able to drink could have severe pneumonia or bronchiolitis, sepsis (a bacterial infection of the bloodstream, also called septicaemia), an infection of the brain (meningitis or cerebral malaria), a throat abscess, or other problems. Oxygen, antibiotics and other medicines are life-saving for some of these children.

Convulsions, abnormally sleepy or difficult to wake:

A child with these signs may have severe pneumonia resulting in too little oxygen being taken in (hypoxia), sepsis, cerebral malaria (in areas with falciparum malaria) or meningitis. Meningitis can develop as a complication of pneumonia, or it can occur on its own.

Stridor in calm child:

If a child has stridor when calm, the child may be in danger of a life-threatening obstruction of the airway from swelling of the larynx, trachea or epiglottis.

Severe malnutrition:

A severely malnourished child is at high risk of developing, and dying from, pneumonia. In addition, the child may not show typical signs of illness.

Treatment

A child who is classified as having very severe disease is *very* ill, and should be referred *urgently* to a hospital:

- Before the child leaves the health centre, you should provide any treatment needed, write a note to the referral hospital, and make sure that the mother is willing and able to take the child to the hospital immediately. (Annex 3 gives a more detailed description of how to refer a child to a hospital.)

- Give the first dose of antibiotic before the child leaves the health centre. You should also treat fever and wheezing, if present.

- If there is falciparum malaria in the area, and the child has any fever or a history of fever with convulsions, is abnormally sleepy or difficult to wake, or is not able to drink, he or she should also receive an antimalarial. These signs indicate that the child may have cerebral malaria, which can be fatal if it is not treated quickly. Follow the guidelines of your national malaria programme for treatment of this condition.

- If referral is not feasible, follow the recommendations in Annex 4.

Management of a child aged 2 months up to 5 years who is classified as having very severe disease is summarized on the chart below.

Locate this section on the fold-out chart.

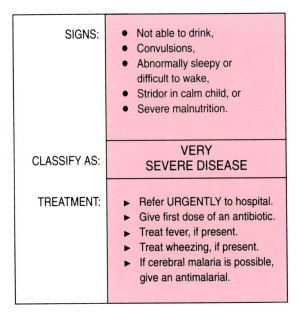

SIGNS:	• Not able to drink, • Convulsions, • Abnormally sleepy or difficult to wake, • Stridor in calm child, or • Severe malnutrition.
CLASSIFY AS:	**VERY SEVERE DISEASE**
TREATMENT:	▶ Refer URGENTLY to hospital. ▶ Give first dose of an antibiotic. ▶ Treat fever, if present. ▶ Treat wheezing, if present. ▶ If cerebral malaria is possible, give an antimalarial.

Deciding if the child has pneumonia

If you identified a danger sign in the preceding step, you have already classified the child's illness, and you know to refer the child urgently. Do *not* try to determine if the child also has pneumonia. *Each child should be put in a single classification.* However, if you did *not* identify a danger sign, the next step is to use the clinical information from the assessment to decide:

• Does the child have pneumonia?
Ask this question only about children who do not have danger signs. The child without danger signs is classified as having either:

— severe pneumonia,
— pneumonia (not severe), or
— no pneumonia: cough or cold.

On the following pages is a description of each of these classifications. Read this information carefully so that you know what signs to look for. The most important signs to consider when deciding if the child has pneumonia are:

— the child's breathing rate, and
— whether or not there is chest indrawing.

Refer to the chart to find the one box that matches the child's signs. By first deciding if the child should be classified as having very severe disease, and then deciding if the child has pneumonia, you will be less likely to overlook an important sign and treat a very sick child incorrectly.

Locate the signs and classifications of pneumonia in the boxes below. Then find these boxes on the fold-out chart.

SIGNS:	• Chest indrawing. [If also recurrent wheezing, go directly to ▶ **Treat Wheezing**]	• **No** chest indrawing, and • **Fast breathing** (**50** per minute or more if child 2 months up to 12 months; **40** per minute or more if child 12 months up to 5 years).	• **No** chest indrawing and • **No** fast breathing (Less than **50** per minute if child 2 months up to 12 months; Less than **40** per minute if child 12 months up to 5 years).
CLASSIFY AS:	**SEVERE PNEUMONIA**	**PNEUMONIA**	**NO PNEUMONIA: COUGH OR COLD**
TREATMENT:	▶ Refer URGENTLY to hospital. ▶ Give first dose of an antibiotic. ▶ Treat fever, if present. ▶ Treat wheezing, if present. (If referral is not feasible, treat with an antibiotic and follow closely.)	▶ Advise mother to give home care. ▶ Give an antibiotic. ▶ Treat fever, if present. ▶ Treat wheezing, if present. ▶ Advise mother to return with child in 2 days for reassessment, or earlier if the child is getting worse.	▶ If coughing more than 30 days, refer for assessment. ▶ Assess and treat ear problem or sore throat, if present (see chart). ▶ Assess and treat other problems. ▶ Advise mother to give home care. ▶ Treat fever, if present. ▶ Treat wheezing, if present.

Severe pneumonia

> **A child with:**
> *chest indrawing*
> **is classified as having *severe pneumonia***

A child with chest indrawing usually has severe pneumonia. Chest indrawing occurs when the lungs become stiff and the effort required to breathe in is much greater than normal.

A child with chest indrawing may not have fast breathing. If the child becomes tired, and if the effort needed to expand the lungs is too great, then the breathing slows down. Therefore, chest indrawing may be the *only* sign that the child has severe pneumonia. A child with chest indrawing is at higher risk of death from pneumonia than the child with fast breathing without chest indrawing.

A child classified as having severe pneumonia might also have other signs:

- Nasal flaring, when the nose widens as the child breathes in.
- Grunting, the short sounds made with the voice when the child has difficulty breathing.
- Cyanosis, a dark bluish or purplish coloration of the skin, caused by hypoxia. If the tongue is cyanosed, the child should be given oxygen.

A child with any of these other signs will also have chest indrawing or danger signs of very severe disease. Thus, it is not necessary to teach these other possible signs to health workers. However, if health workers already recognize them, the signs help support a classification of severe pneumonia.

Some children with chest indrawing also have wheezing. Children who have chest indrawing and a *first episode* of wheezing often have severe pneumonia. However, children with chest indrawing and *recurrent* wheezing most often do not have severe pneumonia. Chest indrawing in these children is caused by the recurrent wheezing (asthma), rather than severe pneumonia. Therefore, they must be managed differently. They must be assessed further before you can decide what kind of treatment is needed. Instructions for carrying out this assessment are described in Chapter 5, and are summarized in the box, "Treat wheezing" on the chart.

Treatment

A child who is classified as having severe pneumonia should be referred urgently to a hospital (see Annex 3):

- The child should receive the first dose of antibiotic.
- Fever and wheezing, if present, should be treated.

Management of the child classified as having severe pneumonia is summarized on the chart below.

SIGNS:	• Chest indrawing. [If also recurrent wheezing, go directly to ▶ ***Treat Wheezing***]
CLASSIFY AS:	**SEVERE PNEUMONIA**
TREATMENT:	▶ Refer URGENTLY to hospital. ▶ Give first dose of an antibiotic. ▶ Treat fever, if present. ▶ Treat wheezing, if present. (If referral is not feasible, treat with an antibiotic and follow closely.)

How to give an antibiotic and how to treat fever and wheezing are described in detail in Chapter 5.

If referral is not feasible, see the recommendations in Annex 4.

Pneumonia (not severe)

> **A child who has:**
>
> **no chest indrawing**
> **and**
> **fast breathing**
> **(50 per minute or more if 2 months up to 12 months;**
> **40 per minute or more if 12 months up to 5 years)**
> **is classified as having *pneumonia* (not severe).**

A child with fast breathing and *no* chest indrawing is classified as having pneumonia (not severe). Most children with pneumonia are not classified as having severe pneumonia, especially if they are brought early for treatment.

Treatment

The child classified as having pneumonia (not severe) should be treated at home with an antibiotic:

- Infections of the respiratory tract may be caused by viruses or bacteria.

  Bacteria are killed by antibiotics. In developing countries, pneumonia is often caused by bacteria. Antibiotic treatment can thus prevent many deaths from pneumonia if given early enough in the infection.

  Antibiotics do not kill viruses. Although pneumonia can be caused by a virus, there is no reliable way to distinguish viral from bacterial pneumonia. For this reason, children should be given an antibiotic whenever they have signs of pneumonia.

- The mother should be given instructions on home care, including when to return if the child is getting worse and how to give the antibiotic.

- She should also be advised to return with the child in 2 days (48 hours) for reassessment, or earlier if any of the following signs occur:

  — the child's breathing becomes more difficult or faster,
  — the child is not able to drink, or
  — the child becomes sicker.

- Reassessment of children on antibiotic therapy is very important because a few children will not respond to the antibiotic.

Management of the child who is classified as having pneumonia (not severe) is summarized on the chart below.

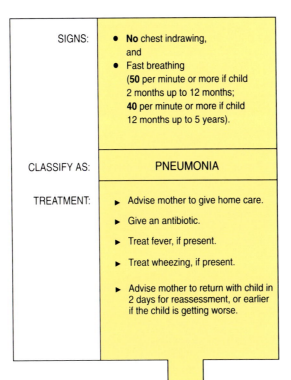

SIGNS:	• **No** chest indrawing, and • Fast breathing (**50** per minute or more if child 2 months up to 12 months; **40** per minute or more if child 12 months up to 5 years).
CLASSIFY AS:	**PNEUMONIA**
TREATMENT:	► Advise mother to give home care. ► Give an antibiotic. ► Treat fever, if present. ► Treat wheezing, if present. ► Advise mother to return with child in 2 days for reassessment, or earlier if the child is getting worse.

	Reassess in 2 days a child who is taking an antibiotic for pneumonia:		
	WORSE	**THE SAME**	**IMPROVING**
SIGNS:	• Not able to drink. • Has chest indrawing. • Has other danger signs.		• Breathing slower. • Less fever. • Eating better.
TREATMENT:	► Refer URGENTLY to hospital.	► Change antibiotic or Refer.	► Finish 5 days of antibiotic.

Advice on home care, how to give an antibiotic, how to treat fever and wheezing, and the reassessment of the child on antibiotic therapy are described in detail in Chapter 5.

No pneumonia: cough or cold

> **A child who has:**
> *no chest indrawing*
> **and**
> *no fast breathing*
> *(less than 50 per minute if 2 months up to 12 months;*
> *less than 40 per minute if 12 months up to 5 years)*
> **is classified as having *no pneumonia: cough or cold*.**

Most children with a cough or difficult breathing do not have any danger signs or signs of pneumonia (chest indrawing or fast breathing). These children have a simple cough or cold. They are classified as having no pneumonia: cough or cold.

Treatment

Treat the child who is classified as having no pneumonia: cough or cold by advising the mother to give home care:

- *Do not give an antibiotic* to a child with a cough or cold who has no signs of pneumonia. *It will not relieve the symptoms or prevent the cold from developing into pneumonia.*

- Although the child with a cough or cold does not need an antibiotic, the mother has brought the child to the clinic because of an illness that concerns her. These concerns need to be addressed and advice given on good home care. In particular, she must know to watch for signs of pneumonia and to return if these develop. Advising the mother on good home care for the child with a simple cough or cold will help ensure that she will bring the child back to the clinic for further treatment if the child does develop pneumonia.

However, some children with a cough or cold have additional problems that you must consider:

- Normally a child with a cold will get better within 1–2 weeks. However, a child with a chronic cough (lasting more than 30 days) may have tuberculosis,[1] asthma, whooping cough or another problem. Refer the child with a chronic cough to a hospital for further assessment.

SIGNS:	• **No** chest indrawing and • **No** fast breathing (Less than **50** per minute if child 2 months up to 12 months; Less than **40** per minute if child 12 months up to 5 years).
CLASSIFY AS:	**NO PNEUMONIA: COUGH OR COLD**
TREATMENT:	▶ If coughing more than 30 days, refer for assessment. ▶ Assess and treat ear problem or sore throat, if present (see chart). ▶ Assess and treat other problems. ▶ Advise mother to give home care. ▶ Treat fever, if present. ▶ Treat wheezing, if present.

---

[1] Tuberculosis should be suspected if anyone in the family has the disease, or if the child is malnourished, has a swelling in the neck or under the arm, or has continuing fevers. Children with suspected tuberculosis should be referred for a chest X-ray and assessment by a doctor familiar with childhood tuberculosis. Consult your national tuberculosis control programme.

- If the child has an ear problem (ear pain or pus draining from the ear) or a sore throat, assess the child further. See Chapters 6 and 7 and the fold-out chart, "Management of the Child with an Ear Problem or Sore Throat" at the back of this book.

- Assess and treat other problems such as diarrhoea or skin problems. Check the child's immunization status and immunize if needed.

- Treat fever and wheezing, if present (see Chapter 5).

Management of the child who is classified as having no pneumonia: cough or cold is summarized on the chart on page 22.

Advice on home care, and how to treat fever and wheezing are described in Chapter 5.

This chapter has described the four classifications of illness for a child aged 2 months up to 5 years, and how to decide in which classification a child belongs. The examples below illustrate how to use the case management chart to classify a child's illness, and how to avoid missing important signs.

Examples

1. Karana is 2 years old. Her mother brought her to the health centre because she had a cough and runny nose. After completing the assessment, the health worker learned that Karana had a slight fever (38.5 °C), but no other signs of illness.

   The health worker looked at the case management chart, "Management of the Child with Cough or Difficult Breathing". Using the boxes for the child aged 2 months up to 5 years:

   - He first asked if Karana had any danger signs, and compared her signs with the signs that correspond to the classification, very severe disease. None of her signs were listed there, so he did not classify her as having very severe disease.

   - Next, he asked himself if she had pneumonia. Karana had neither chest indrawing nor fast breathing. Therefore, the health worker classified Karana as having no pneumonia: cough or cold.

2. Babu's mother brought him to the health centre because he had difficulty breathing. After completing the assessment, the health worker learned that 18-month-old Babu was not able to drink and had stridor when calm. He had chest indrawing, but did not have fast breathing (35 times per minute).

   The health worker looked at the case management chart, "Management of the Child with Cough or Difficult Breathing". Then, using the boxes for the child aged 2 months up to 5 years:

   - She first asked if Babu had any danger signs, and compared Babu's signs with the signs that correspond to the classification, very severe disease. Since Babu had two of the danger signs listed (not able to drink and stridor when calm), the health worker classified him as having very severe disease.

- Even though Babu also had chest indrawing, the health worker did not use this sign to classify Babu's illness. Since each child should only be classified for one disease, the health worker stopped trying to classify the illness as soon as she decided that Babu had very severe disease.

3. Mohammed is 6 months old. His mother brought him to the health centre because he had been coughing for 2 days. After completing the assessment, the health worker learned that Mohammed was abnormally sleepy and difficult to wake, and that he had fast breathing (58 times per minute).

The health worker looked at the case management chart, "Management of the Child with Cough or Difficult Breathing". Using the boxes for the child aged 2 months up to 5 years, he:

- Focused immediately on the fact that Mohammed had fast breathing but no chest indrawing, and classified him as having pneumonia (not severe).

Fortunately, the health centre supervisor noticed that Mohammed was being treated for pneumonia (not severe), even though he also had the danger sign, abnormally sleepy and difficult to wake. The supervisor reminded the health worker that it is very important to first compare the child's signs of illness with the signs that correspond to the classification, very severe disease, to ensure that danger signs are not overlooked. The supervisor then classified Mohammed as having very severe disease, and referred him immediately to a hospital.

Summary review: classifying the illness of the child aged 2 months up to 5 years

Very severe disease

A child with *any danger sign* is classified as having very severe disease. The danger signs are:

- Not able to drink
- Convulsions
- Abnormally sleepy or difficult to wake
- Stridor when calm
- Severe malnutrition.

A child who is classified as having very severe disease should be referred urgently to a hospital.

Severe pneumonia

A child with *chest indrawing* is classified as having severe pneumonia. The child should be referred urgently to a hospital.

However, children with both chest indrawing and recurrent wheezing may have asthma, rather than severe pneumonia. These children are managed differently (see Chapter 5).

Pneumonia (not severe)

A child with *fast breathing and no chest indrawing* is classified as having pneumonia (not severe). The cut-off for fast breathing is:

— 50 times per minute or more if the child is aged 2 months up to 12 months, or
— 40 times per minute or more if the child is aged 12 months up to 5 years.

Children classified as having pneumonia (not severe) should be given antibiotics and home care. The mother should be told to bring the child back after 2 days for reassessment, or earlier if the child worsens.

No pneumonia: cough or cold

A child who does *not have chest indrawing or fast breathing* is classified as having no pneumonia: cough or cold.

Children classified as having no pneumonia: cough or cold should be given home care. They should not be given antibiotics.

Essential skills and knowledge

By the end of this chapter, you should be able to do the following:

- Classify the illness of the child aged 2 months up to 5 years with cough or difficult breathing, based on signs found during the assessment.

Classification	Corresponding signs
Very severe disease	Not able to drink, convulsions, abnormally sleepy or difficult to wake, stridor when calm, or severe malnutrition
Severe pneumonia	Chest indrawing
Pneumonia	No chest indrawing, and fast breathing
No pneumonia: cough or cold	No chest indrawing, and no fast breathing

- Select appropriate treatment for the child aged 2 months up to 5 years based on the above classifications: refer, give an antibiotic, or advise the mother to give home care.

CHAPTER 4

Classifying the illness of the young infant (aged less than 2 months)

This chapter describes how to classify the illness of the young infant with cough or difficult breathing, and identify the appropriate treatment plan. The process is similar to the one described in the previous chapter for the child aged 2 months up to 5 years.

Young infants have special characteristics that must be considered when their illness is classified. They can become sick and die very quickly from serious bacterial infections, are much less likely to cough with pneumonia, and frequently have only non-specific signs such as poor feeding, fever or low body temperature. Further, mild chest indrawing is normal in young infants because their chest wall bones are soft.

The presence of these characteristics means that the health worker will assess, classify and treat young infants differently from older children. The differences between the two age groups are presented in detail in this chapter. Briefly, the most important differences are:

- Some of the danger signs are different. In a young infant, danger signs include "stopped feeding well", "fever or low body temperature", and "wheezing". The sign "severe malnutrition" is not a danger sign in young infants, although it is in older children.

- A young infant must have *severe* chest indrawing to be classified as having severe pneumonia. A child aged 2 months up to 5 years is classified as having severe pneumonia if there is *any* chest indrawing that is clearly visible.

- The cut-off for fast breathing is different. A young infant has fast breathing when he or she is breathing 60 times per minute or more. The cut-offs for fast breathing in children aged 2 months up to 5 years are 50 times per minute or more if the children are aged 2 months up to 12 months, or 40 times per minute or more if they are aged 12 months up to 5 years.

- Any pneumonia in young infants is considered to be severe. Young infants with pneumonia should be referred immediately to a hospital. Older children can be classified as having "pneumonia" (which can be treated at home with an antibiotic) or "severe pneumonia" (in which case they should be referred urgently to a hospital).

Refer to the fold-out case management chart and find the boxes under the heading, "Classify the illness".

Note that the boxes in this section are either red or green. Each colour refers to one of the two treatment plans.

- Red means, "refer urgently to hospital".
- Green means, "give home care".

The colour of the boxes will help you to determine quickly the severity of the illness and the appropriate treatment plan.

Then, find the subheading, "The young infant age less than 2 months".

The boxes below this subheading should be used to classify the illness of a young infant. These boxes are reproduced below.

THE YOUNG INFANT
AGE LESS THAN 2 MONTHS

SIGNS:	• Stopped feeding well, • Convulsions, • Abnormally sleepy or difficult to wake, • Stridor in calm child, • Wheezing, or • Fever or low body temperature.
CLASSIFY AS:	**VERY SEVERE DISEASE**
TREATMENT:	▶ Refer URGENTLY to hospital. ▶ Keep young infant warm. ▶ Give first dose of an antibiotic.

SIGNS:	• Severe chest indrawing, or • Fast breathing (60 per minute or MORE).	• **No** severe chest indrawing, and • **No** fast breathing (LESS than 60 per minute).
CLASSIFY AS:	**SEVERE PNEUMONIA**	**NO PNEUMONIA: COUGH OR COLD**

TREATMENT:	▶ Refer URGENTLY to hospital.
	
	▶ Keep young infant warm.
	
	▶ Give first dose of an antibiotic.
	
	(If referral is not feasible, treat with an antibiotic and follow closely.)
		▶ Advise mother to give the following home care:
		  ▶ Keep young infant warm.
		  ▶ Breast-feed frequently.
		  ▶ Clear nose if it interferes with feeding.
		  ▶ Return quickly if:
		    ▶ Breathing becomes difficult.
		    ▶ Breathing becomes fast.
		    ▶ Feeding becomes a problem.
		    ▶ The young infant becomes sicker.

Deciding if the young infant has very severe disease

As stated earlier, there are three classifications of illness for a young infant with a cough or difficult breathing: very severe disease, severe pneumonia, and no pneumonia: cough or cold. To classify the young infant's illness, you should follow the steps as they are presented in this chapter. The first step is to decide if the young infant should be classified as having very severe disease.

You can decide if a young infant should be classified as having very severe disease by using the clinical information from the assessment to determine whether the young infant has a "danger sign". *Ask this question about every young infant with a cough or difficult breathing:*

- Does the child have danger signs?

A young infant with:
any danger sign
is classified as having *very severe disease*

A young infant with a danger sign may be at high risk of dying. It is difficult to distinguish between infections such as pneumonia, sepsis and meningitis in such an infant. However, it is not necessary to make this distinction. You need only to recognize the danger signs and know that the young infant has very severe disease.

Some of the danger signs in children aged 2 months up to 5 years are also danger signs in young infants:

Convulsions, abnormally sleepy or difficult to wake:	A young infant with these signs may have hypoxia, sepsis or meningitis. (Malaria infection is unusual in children of this age, so antimalarial treatment for possible cerebral malaria is not advised.)
Stridor when calm:	Infections causing stridor (e.g. diphtheria, bacterial tracheitis, measles or epiglottitis) are rare in young infants. A young infant who has stridor when calm should be classified as having very severe disease.

However, some signs are danger signs in young infants, but not in older children:

Stopped feeding well:	A young infant who stops feeding well (that is, takes less than half of the usual amount of milk) may have a serious infection and should be classified as having very severe disease.[1]
Wheezing:	Wheezing is uncommon in young infants, and is often associated with hypoxia.

---

[1] Older children with respiratory infections often stop feeding well, but this is not a danger sign for them. The danger sign in the older child is "not able to drink".

Fever or low body temperature: Fever (38 °C or more) is uncommon in young infants and more often means a serious bacterial infection than in older children. In addition, fever may be the only sign of a serious bacterial infection. In young infants an infection may cause the body temperature to drop below 35.5 °C (hypothermia).

Treatment

A young infant who is classified as having very severe disease should be referred *urgently* to a hospital for treatment (see Annex 3):

- Write a note to the referral hospital, and make sure that the mother is willing and able to take the young infant to the hospital immediately.
- Give the first dose of antibiotic.
- It is very important to keep the young infant warm. Low temperature alone can kill young infants. Wrapping the young infant next to the mother is a good way to keep the infant warm during the journey to the hospital.

Management of the young infant who is classified as having very severe disease is summarized in the chart below.

SIGNS:	• Stopped feeding well, • Convulsions, • Abnormally sleepy or difficult to wake, • Stridor in calm child, • Wheezing, or • Fever or low body temperature.
CLASSIFY AS:	**VERY SEVERE DISEASE**
TREATMENT:	► Refer URGENTLY to hospital. ► Keep young infant warm. ► Give first dose of an antibiotic.

Deciding if the young infant has pneumonia

If you have identified a danger sign in the preceding step, you have already classified the young infant's illness, and you know to refer the young infant urgently to a hospital. Do not also try to determine if the young infant has pneumonia. *Each young infant should be put in a single classification.*

However, if you did not identify a danger sign, use the clinical information from the assessment to decide:

• Does the child have pneumonia?

Ask this question only about young infants who do not have any danger signs. The young infant without danger signs has either:

— Severe pneumonia, or
— No pneumonia: cough or cold.

Note that the classification pneumonia (not severe) is not included as it was for older children. Young infants can become sick and die very quickly from serious bacterial infections such as pneumonia, sepsis and meningitis. Therefore, any young infant who has a sign of pneumonia is classified as having severe pneumonia.

On the following pages is a description of the two classifications that apply to young infants. Read this information carefully so that you know what signs to look for. The most important signs to consider when deciding if the young infant has pneumonia are:

— the breathing rate, and
— whether or not there is severe chest indrawing.

Refer to the case management chart to find the one box that matches the young infant's signs. By first deciding if the young infant should be classified as having very severe disease, and then deciding if he or she has pneumonia, you will be less likely to overlook an important sign and treat a very sick young infant incorrectly.

Locate the signs of pneumonia and the classifications of severe pneumonia and no pneumonia: cough or cold in the boxes below. Then find these boxes on the fold-out case management chart.

SIGNS:	• Severe chest indrawing, or • Fast breathing (60 per minute or MORE).	• **No** severe chest indrawing, and • **No** fast breathing (LESS than 60 per minute).
CLASSIFY AS:	**SEVERE PNEUMONIA**	**NO PNEUMONIA: COUGH OR COLD**

TREATMENT:	▶ Refer URGENTLY to hospital.
	
	▶ Keep young infant warm.
	
	▶ Give first dose of an antibiotic.
	
	(If referral is not feasible, treat with an antibiotic and follow closely.)
		▶ Advise mother to give the following home care:
		  ▶ Keep young infant warm.
		  ▶ Breast-feed frequently.
		  ▶ Clear nose if it interferes with feeding.
		  ▶ Return quickly if:
		    ▶ Breathing becomes difficult.
		    ▶ Breathing becomes fast.
		    ▶ Feeding becomes a problem.
		    ▶ The young infant becomes sicker.

Severe pneumonia

A young infant who has:
fast breathing
(60 times per minute or more),
or
severe chest indrawing
is classified as having *severe pneumonia*

Young infants usually breathe faster than older children. The breathing rate of a healthy young infant is commonly more than 50 breaths per minute. Therefore, a rate of 60 breaths per minute or more is used to identify fast breathing in a young infant.

Mild chest indrawing is normal in young infants because their chest wall bones are soft. However, *severe* chest indrawing (very deep and easy to see) is a sign of pneumonia. Since pneumonia in a young infant can progress very rapidly to death, all pneumonia is considered severe in this age group.

Treatment

A young infant who is classified as having severe pneumonia should be referred *urgently* to a hospital (see Annex 3). The young infant needs antibiotics by injection. Home care with antibiotics is much less effective and is not recommended.

SIGNS:	• Severe chest indrawing, or • Fast breathing (60 per minute or MORE).
CLASSIFY AS:	**SEVERE PNEUMONIA**
TREATMENT:	▶ Refer URGENTLY to hospital. ▶ Keep young infant warm. ▶ Give first dose of an antibiotic. (If referral is not feasible, treat with an antibiotic and follow closely.)

- Write a note to the referral hospital, and make sure that the mother is willing and able to take the young infant to the hospital immediately.
- Give the first dose of antibiotic.
- Keeping a sick young infant warm is very important. Low temperature alone can kill young infants. Wrapping the young infant next to the mother is a good way to keep the infant warm during the journey to the hospital.

Management of the young infant who is classified as having severe pneumonia is summarized in the chart on page 31. If referral is not feasible, see Annex 4.

No pneumonia: cough or cold

> **A young infant who has:**
> **no fast breathing**
> **(less than 60 times per minute),**
> **and**
> **no severe chest indrawing or danger signs**
> **is classified as having *no pneumonia: cough or cold***

Young infants who have neither fast breathing nor severe chest indrawing, and have no other signs of very severe disease, do not have pneumonia. They have a simple cough or cold.

Treatment

The young infant who does not have signs of pneumonia (or danger signs) can be treated at home without antibiotics. Advise the mother to give the following home care:

- Keep the young infant warm.
- Breast-feed frequently.
- Clear the young infant's nose if it interferes with feeding.

A young infant can become very sick *very quickly*. Therefore, tell the mother to bring the young infant back to the health centre immediately if:

- Breathing becomes difficult.
- Breathing becomes fast.
- Feeding becomes a problem.
- The young infant becomes sicker.

Management of the young infant who is classified as having no pneumonia: cough or cold is summarized in the chart below.

This chapter has described the three classifications of illness for a young infant with a cough or difficult breathing. The examples below illustrate how to use the case management chart to classify the young infant's illness, and how to avoid missing important signs.

SIGNS:	• **No** severe chest indrawing, and • **No** fast breathing (LESS than 60 per minute).
CLASSIFY AS:	NO PNEUMONIA: COUGH OR COLD

TREATMENT:	▶ Advise mother to give the following home care:
	  ▶ Keep young infant warm.
	  ▶ Breast-feed frequently.
	  ▶ Clear nose if it interferes with feeding.
	  ▶ Return quickly if:
	    ▶ Breathing becomes difficult.
	    ▶ Breathing becomes fast.
	    ▶ Feeding becomes a problem.
	    ▶ The young infant becomes sicker.

Examples

1. Sala is 14 days old. His mother brought him to the health centre because he was breathing in an unusual manner. After completing the assessment, the health worker learned that Sala had fast breathing (65 times per minute on the first count, and 72 times per minute on the second count). Sala also had mild, but not severe, chest indrawing.

   The health worker looked at the case management chart, "Management of the Child with Cough or Difficult Breathing". Then, using the boxes for the young infant aged less than 2 months:

   • She first asked herself if Sala had any danger signs, and compared his signs with the signs that correspond to the classification, very severe disease. None of his signs were listed there, so the health worker did not classify Sala as having very severe disease.

   • Then, she asked herself if Sala had pneumonia. Sala had fast breathing, therefore the health worker classified him as having severe pneumonia.

2. Abebech is 6 weeks old. Her mother brought her to the health centre because she was coughing and seemed sick. After completing the assessment, the health worker learned that Abebech had stopped feeding well (she had taken less than half of her usual amount of breast milk), but had no other signs of illness.

   The health worker looked at the case management chart, "Management of the Child with Cough or Difficult Breathing". Then, using the boxes for the young infant aged less than 2 months, he:

- Immediately focused on the fact that Abebech did not have fast breathing or chest indrawing, and classified her as having no pneumonia: cough or cold.

Fortunately, the mother returned the next day because Abebech seemed worse. A more experienced health worker saw that Abebech had stopped feeding well, classified her as having very severe disease, and referred her urgently to a hospital. He reminded the first health worker that it is very important to first compare the young infant's signs of illness with the signs that correspond to the classification, very severe disease, so that danger signs (such as stopped feeding well) are not overlooked.

Summary review: classifying the illness of the young infant

Very severe disease

A young infant with *any danger sign* is classified as having very severe disease. The danger signs are:

- Stopped feeding well
- Convulsions
- Abnormally sleepy or difficult to wake
- Stridor when calm
- Wheezing
- Fever or low body temperature.

Young infants classified as having very severe disease should be referred *urgently* to a hospital.

Severe pneumonia

A young infant who has *fast breathing* (60 times per minute or more) *or severe chest indrawing* is classified as having severe pneumonia.

Young infants classified as having severe pneumonia should be referred *urgently* to a hospital.

No pneumonia: cough or cold

A young infant who is *breathing less than 60 times per minute*, and has *no severe chest indrawing or danger signs*, is classified as having no pneumonia: cough or cold.

Mothers of young infants classified as having no pneumonia: cough or cold should be told to give home care, and to return to the health centre immediately if the young infant's condition worsens, breathing becomes difficult or fast, or feeding becomes a problem.

Antibiotics should not be given to young infants in this classification.

Essential skills and knowledge

By the end of this chapter, you should be able to do the following:

- Classify the illness of a young infant with cough or difficult breathing based on signs found during the assessment.

Classification	Corresponding signs
Very severe disease	Stopped feeding well, convulsions, abnormally sleepy or difficult to wake, stridor when calm, wheezing, fever or low body temperature
Severe pneumonia	Fast breathing (60 times per minute or more) or severe chest indrawing
No pneumonia: cough or cold	No fast breathing (less than 60 times per minute), and no severe chest indrawing or danger signs

- Select appropriate treatment for the young infant based on the above classification: refer, or advise the mother to give home care.

CHAPTER 5
Treatment instructions

The two previous chapters described how to classify the illness of a child or young infant with cough or difficult breathing and identify the appropriate treatment for each classification. This chapter describes how to provide each of these treatments.

The treatments include:

- Give an antibiotic.
- Advise the mother to give home care.
- Treat fever.[1]
- Treat wheezing.[1]

Refer to the fold-out chart and find the heading, "Treatment instructions". Then look at the boxes underneath this heading, and find the box that matches each of the four treatments listed above. Use these boxes when treating a child with a respiratory infection.

Give an antibiotic

WHO recommends treating pneumonia by giving *one* of the following antibiotics for 5 days:

— co-trimoxazole,[2]
— amoxycillin,[3]   } (in tablet or syrup form)
— ampicillin, or
— procaine penicillin[4,5] (by daily intramuscular injection).

You need to learn how to give only the antibiotic(s) used in your health centre. The instructions presented here are for giving an oral antibiotic.

If the child cannot take an oral antibiotic (e.g. if the child is unable to drink or will not wake up), however, you will need to give a parenteral antibiotic, such as procaine penicillin. If you are unable to give parenteral antibiotics, refer the child as quickly as possible without giving the first dose.

---

[1] Fever and wheezing are danger signs in young infants. Young infants with these signs are classified as having very severe disease and should be referred urgently to a hospital.
[2] INN = trimethoprim–sulfamethoxazole.
[3] INN = amoxicillin.
[4] INN = procaine benzylpenicillin.
[5] WHO does not recommend using either benzathine benzylpenicillin or oral phenoxymethylpenicillin (penicillin V) for treatment of pneumonia.

> *Cautions about giving an antibiotic:*
>
> - *Do not give co-trimoxazole to a baby with jaundice, or to a premature baby less than one month old.*
> - *Do not give amoxycillin, ampicillin, procaine penicillin, benzathine penicillin or phenoxymethylpenicillin if the child has a history of breathing problems or anaphylaxis (allergic reaction) after treatment with penicillin.*

Give the first dose of the antibiotic

The child needs to receive the first dose of the antibiotic in the health centre, before being referred to a hospital or sent home to continue treatment. (If the referral time is less than an hour, such as in an urban area, it may not be necessary to give the first dose at the health centre.) If the child is to be treated at home by the mother, you should use this opportunity to show her how to give the antibiotic.

The steps in giving an antibiotic in tablet (or syrup) form are as follows:

1. Decide the correct dose of antibiotic to give.

   - Check the strength in milligrams per tablet (or per 5 ml of syrup) written on the package.
   - Weigh the child. If a scale is not available, use the child's age to determine the dose.
   - Use the table on the bottom of the case management chart (reproduced on the next page) to determine the dose, based on the strength of the tablet (or syrup) and the age or weight of the child.

   Example: To treat an 11-month-old child with paediatric co-trimoxazole tablets

   ---

   - Check to make sure the tablets contain 20 mg of trimethoprim and 100 mg of sulfamethoxazole (paediatric tablets).
   - Use the table to determine a single dose for an 11-month-old child: two paediatric tablets. Co-trimoxazole should be given twice daily, so the total daily dose is four paediatric tablets. Give this amount each day for 5 days.

   The table below shows how to determine the correct dose of antibiotic for children and young infants.

2. Crush the antibiotic tablet in a cup and mix it with a small amount of food to make it easier for the child to swallow. Ask the mother what foods she has at home to mix the powder with, such as porridge. If the child normally takes only breast milk, tell her to express her milk manually and mix it with the powder in a clean bowl.

3. Ask the mother to give the antibiotic to the child, with a spoon, from the cup. The child may accept the antibiotic more easily from the mother. This also gives the mother a chance to try giving the antibiotic once before leaving the health centre. If the child spits out the antibiotic or vomits within 30 minutes of swallowing it, repeat the dose.

▶ *Give an Antibiotic*

▸ Give first dose of antibiotic in clinic.

▸ Instruct mother on how to give the antibiotic for five days at home (or to return to clinic for daily procaine penicillin injection).

AGE or WEIGHT	COTRIMOXAZOLE (trimethoprim + sulphamethoxazole) ▸ Two times daily for 5 days.			AMOXYCILLIN ▸ Three times daily for 5 days.		AMPICILLIN ▸ Four times daily for 5 days.		PROCAINE PENICILLIN ▸ Once daily for 5 days.
	Adult Tablet single strength (80 mg trimethoprim + 400 mg sulphamethoxazole)	Pediatric Tablet (20 mg trimethoprim + 100 mg sulphamethoxazole)	Syrup (40 mg trimethoprim + 200 mg sulphamethoxazole per 5 ml)	Tablet 250 mg	Syrup 125 mg in 5 ml	Tablet 250 mg	Syrup 250 mg in 5 ml	Intramuscular Injection
Less than 2 months (< 5 kg) ✦	1/4*	1*	2.5 ml*	1/4	2.5 ml	1/2	2.5 ml	200,000 units
2 months up to 12 months (6-9 kg)	1/2	2	5 ml	1/2	5 ml	1	5 ml	400,000 units
12 months up to 5 years (10-19 kg)	1	3	7.5 ml	1	10 ml	1	5 ml	800,000 units

✦ Give oral antibiotic for 5 days at home only if referral is not feasible.

* If the child is less than 1 month old, give 1/2 pediatric tablet or 1.25 ml syrup twice daily.
Avoid cotrimoxazole in infants less than one month of age who are premature or jaundiced.

Teach the mother to give the antibiotic at home

1. Explain carefully to the mother *how much* of the antibiotic to give, *how often* to give it, and *when* to give it. Write this information down for her. If she cannot read, draw a simple picture.

2. Give the mother enough antibiotics for 5 days. Explain to the mother that she must:

   • Give the child the antibiotic for 5 days.
   • Finish the 5-day treatment, even if the child seems better.

3. Make sure that the mother understands all the instructions and will be able to carry them out. There are several ways to do this:

   • Ask the mother to repeat the instructions (e.g. the dosage). Then, correct any mistakes that she makes.
   • Ask the mother to demonstrate what she has heard. Then, if necessary, show her again how to do the task correctly.
   • Help the mother plan how she will give the antibiotic on the dosing schedule.
   • Ask her what problems she might have giving the child the antibiotic. Then, help her to find a way of overcoming them. For example, if she is working away from home and will have difficulty giving all the doses, help her identify someone who could care for the child and give the child the antibiotic when she is away.

4. Advise the mother on how to give home care (see page 39).

5. Ask the mother to bring the child back to be reassessed in 2 days, or sooner if the child worsens. You need to reassess the child to see whether the child is improving with the antibiotic.

> Treatment instructions should always end with the mother knowing what to do at home and how to do it

Reassess in 2 days a child who is taking an antibiotic for pneumonia

The mother of any child receiving an antibiotic for pneumonia should bring the child back in 2 days, or sooner if the child worsens. During reassessment, you should follow the same procedures as for assessing a child with cough or difficult breathing for the first time (see Chapter 2).

Use the information about the child's signs to decide whether the child is:

— worse,
— the same, or
— improving.

The child has worsened if he or she has more difficulty breathing, is not able to drink, has chest indrawing, or has other danger signs. Refer the child urgently to a hospital.

The child has improved if he or she is breathing more slowly, has less fever (the fever is lower or has gone completely), or is eating better. The cough may still be present. Tell the mother to finish the 5-day course of antibiotics.

If the child is the same as at the last assessment, ask the mother whether the child has been given the antibiotic. There may have been problems so that the child did not receive any of the antibiotic, or received too low or too infrequent a dose (e.g. the child may have refused it, or it may have been destroyed or lost). If so, this child can be given the same antibiotic again.

If the child received the antibiotic, change the antibiotic (if you have another appropriate antibiotic available for childhood pneumonia). Give the other antibiotic for 5 days (use the table on page 38 to determine the correct dose):

- If the child was taking co-trimoxazole, switch to ampicillin, amoxycillin or procaine penicillin;
- If the child was taking ampicillin, amoxycillin or procaine penicillin, switch to co-trimoxazole.

If you do not have another appropriate antibiotic available, refer the child to a hospital.

Advise the mother to give home care

Home care is very important for a child with an acute respiratory infection, and most children you manage will be treated with it. Good home care means that the mother will:

- Feed the child to prevent weight loss. Weight loss can contribute to malnutrition.
- Increase the amount of fluids in the child's diet to prevent dehydration. Dehydration can weaken the child and make the child even more sick.
- Soothe the child's sore throat and relieve the cough with a safe remedy.
- Most important: watch for signs that the child is getting worse and return quickly to the health centre if they occur.

It is your responsibility to teach the mother how to provide home care, and to ensure that she understands why it is important. If the child has a simple cough or cold, explain why the child will not get an antibiotic. Thank the mother for bringing the child to the health centre, so she is more likely to return if the child seems worse.

Home care advice for mothers of children aged 2 months up to 5 years[1] is summarized on the chart below, and described in the pages that follow.

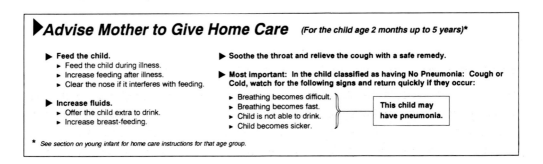

Feed the child

● *Feed the child during illness.*
Children older than 4–6 months of age should be given nutrient-rich and energy-rich foods.[2] Depending on the child's age, these should be mixtures of cereals and vegetables or pulses (e.g. beans), or mixtures of cereals and meat or fish. Increase the energy content of the food by adding vegetable oil. Also give the child dairy products and eggs, if available. Encourage the child to eat as much as he or she wants. If the child is less than 4 months old or has not started taking soft foods, encourage the mother to breast-feed frequently.

● *Increase feeding after illness.*
Children often eat less while they are ill. Therefore, after the respiratory infection is over, *give one extra meal each day for a week*, or until the child has regained normal weight. This will help the child regain normal health and prevent malnutrition. Malnutrition increases the chance that the next time the child gets a respiratory infection or diarrhoea, he or she will become more seriously ill.

● *Clear the nose if it interferes with feeding.*
If the child is not feeding well because of a blocked nose, clear it using a soft cloth. If the nose is blocked by dry or thick, sticky mucus, salted water can be put in the nose (using a moistened wick) to help soften the mucus. Do not use nose drops in young infants.

See Annex 2 for advice on feeding children with measles or pertussis.

Increase fluids

● *Offer the child extra to drink.*
Children with a respiratory infection can lose more fluids than usual, especially when they have a fever. Tell the mother to give the child more fluids than usual. Examples of suitable

---

[1] Home care advice for mothers of young infants is found on pages 32 and 33.
[2] These foods are also recommended for weaning, for children with malnutrition, and for feeding during and after diarrhoea. Health workers should be familiar with acceptable local recipes that are rich in energy and nutrients, composed of readily available ingredients, and compatible with existing practices and beliefs regarding feeding of children during health and illness.

fluids are: breast milk, water, formula or cow's milk, rice water or water in which other cereals have been cooked, home-made soups, yoghurt-based drinks, and fresh fruit juices.

- *Increase breast-feeding.*
  If the child is exclusively breast-fed, advise the mother to breast-feed more frequently than usual.

Soothe the throat and relieve the cough with a safe remedy

The mother can soothe the child's throat and relieve the cough by giving the child tea sweetened with sugar or honey or a safe, home-made cough syrup or soothing remedy.[1] She can also use a commercial remedy, provided it does not contain any harmful ingredients.[2] However, commercial medicines are often expensive and usually no more effective than home remedies.

Most important! Watch for signs of pneumonia

Instruct the mother of a child classified as having no pneumonia: cough or cold[3] to watch for the following signs, and to bring the child back quickly to the health centre if they occur:

- Breathing becomes difficult.
- Breathing becomes fast.
- The child is not able to drink.
- The child becomes sicker.

Explain to her that if the child has any of these signs, he or she may have a serious illness called pneumonia.

Whenever possible, give the mother a written record of the home care instructions she should follow. Fig. 5 provides an example of a written record that could be given to mothers of children aged 2 months up to 5 years who do not have pneumonia. Note that this record would not be suitable for children of that age with pneumonia, or for young infants.

Treat fever

Fever is common in acute respiratory infections. The method of treating fever in a child aged 2 months up to 5 years will depend on whether the fever is high or low (see Fig. 6).

If the fever is *high* (39 °C or more):[4]

- The child will feel better and eat better if the fever is lowered with paracetamol. It is harder for a child with pneumonia to breathe when he or she has a high fever.

---

[1] Some health centres will provide an effective, soothing remedy for cough.
[2] Health workers should review the common commercial cough and cold remedies, so that they can tell mothers which ones contain potentially harmful ingredients such as atropine, codeine, ethanol, promethazine or high doses of antihistamines, and which are not harmful and may help to relieve symptoms.
[3] Instructions on home care for a child who is classified as having pneumonia (not severe) are described on pages 20 and 21.
[4] The Fahrenheit equivalent for 39 °C is 102.2 °F.

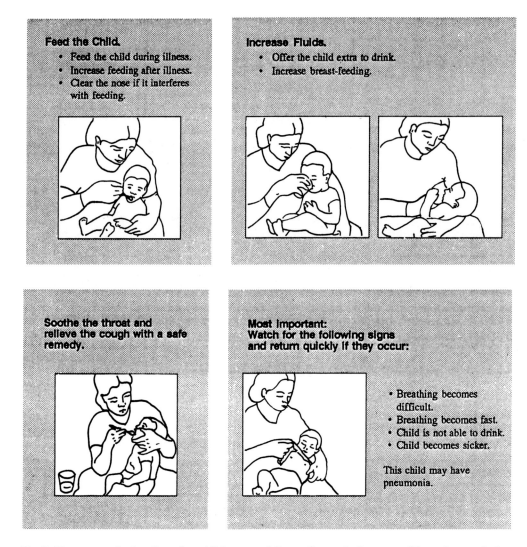

Fig. 5. **Home care instructions for children aged 2 months up to 5 years with acute respiratory infections**

Tell the mother to give the child paracetamol every 6 hours in the appropriate dosage until the child's temperature drops below 39 °C (see the table on page 43 for dosages). Give the mother enough paracetamol for 2 days.

If the fever is *low* (38–39 °C):[1]

• Advise the mother to give the child more fluids than usual. Paracetamol is not needed.

Tell the mother to keep the child with any fever (38 °C or more) lightly clothed. She should not overwrap or overdress the child, since this will make him or her uncomfortable and may make the fever worse.

Children aged 2 months up to 5 years should *not* be given antibiotics if they have fever alone. However, fever is a danger sign in young infants, so young infants with fever should be given a first dose of antibiotic and referred to a hospital. They should not be given paracetamol for fever.

---

[1] The Fahrenheit equivalent for 38 °C is 100.4 °F. These thresholds are based on rectal temperature. The thresholds for axillary temperature readings are approximately 0.5 °C lower.

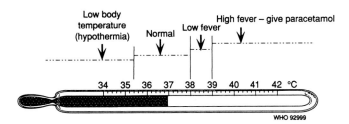

Fig. 6. **Recognizing fever**

Additional comments about fever

In areas with falciparum malaria:

A child who comes to a health centre with cough or difficult breathing *and* a fever (or history of fever) may have malaria. If the infection is not treated quickly, the child may become seriously ill. Therefore, an antimalarial is usually given to treat possible falciparum malaria. In some cases this means that you will give children with pneumonia and a fever (or a history of fever) an

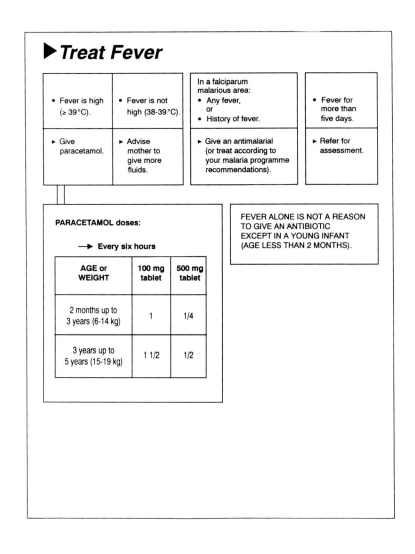

antibiotic for pneumonia *and* an antimalarial for malaria.[1]

If the child has a fever for more than 5 days:

If the child continues to have a fever for more than 5 days, refer the child to a hospital for further assessment.

The steps to follow when treating a fever are summarized in the chart on page 43.

Treat wheezing

This section describes how to treat a child aged 2 months up to 5 years with a first episode of wheezing, and how to assess a child who has recurrent wheezing.

Children with a first episode of wheezing

Use a bronchodilator to treat children with a first episode of wheezing. A bronchodilator[2] is a drug that helps children with wheezing to breathe more easily by opening the air passages of their lungs and relaxing the bronchospasm.

Before giving the bronchodilator, look to see if the child is in respiratory distress. Signs of respiratory distress are:

— the child is uncomfortable,
— the child is obviously not getting enough air into the lungs,
— the child may have difficulty feeding or talking.

This condition can usually be recognized by simple observation. However, most children who wheeze are not in respiratory distress. They are alert and are getting enough air into their lungs.

If the child is in respiratory distress, give a rapid-acting bronchodilator and refer the child immediately to a hospital. The bronchodilator should be given in rapid-acting form so that the child begins to breathe more easily before he or she is referred. (Annex 5 provides a description of how to administer a rapid-acting bronchodilator.)

If you are unable to administer a rapid-acting bronchodilator, give the first dose of an oral bronchodilator (see below), and refer the child immediately to a hospital.

If the child is not in respiratory distress, give an oral bronchodilator (preferably salbutamol) in the appropriate dosage (determined by using the chart on page 46), and show the mother how to give it.

---

[1] In areas with falciparum malaria, co-trimoxazole can be used both as an antibiotic and an antimalarial if it is given for 5 days and if the malaria parasites are sensitive to it. Follow the recommendations of your national malaria control programme.

[2] Salbutamol and epinephrine are two of the most common and effective bronchodilators. Salbutamol is preferred to epinephrine, however, because there is a much lower risk of overdose. Therefore, if available, use salbutamol to treat children who are wheezing.

If the child will be referred for other reasons (e.g. danger signs or chest indrawing), give a single dose of oral salbutamol. If there is no other reason for referral, treat the child based on other signs you see (e.g. fast breathing or fever) and give the mother enough salbutamol for 5 days of treatment. Tell her to give it three times daily.

Children with recurrent wheezing (asthma)

Use a bronchodilator to further assess children with recurrent wheezing (asthma). This assessment will help avoid sending many children to a hospital because you think they have pneumonia, when in fact they have asthma and may not need to be referred.

- Give the bronchodilator in rapid-acting form to all children with recurrent wheezing.[1] (Annex 5 provides instructions on how to administer a rapid-acting bronchodilator.)

- Assess the child's condition 30 minutes later using the table below.

If the child has:	Then:
Respiratory distress or any danger sign	Follow the treatment plan for severe pneumonia or very severe disease.
No respiratory distress and:	
— fast breathing	Follow the treatment plan for pneumonia. Give oral salbutamol in the dosages described in the table on page 46.
— no fast breathing	Follow the treatment plan for no pneumonia: cough or cold. Give oral salbutamol in the dosages described in the table on page 46.

If a child with recurrent wheezing also has a danger sign, you should remember that this child needs *urgent* referral to a hospital. Since the assessment process for recurrent wheezing requires additional time, it may cause an unacceptable delay in referral. You will learn with clinical experience which children with recurrent wheezing and a danger sign should be further assessed with a rapid-acting bronchodilator, and which should be referred without any further assessment.

However, most children with recurrent wheezing have asthma. They may come often to the health centre with wheezing. You will come to recognize these children and treat them promptly with a bronchodilator.

---

[1] If you do not have a rapid-acting bronchodilator, give the child an oral bronchodilator (such as oral salbutamol) instead.

The steps to follow when treating a child with wheezing are summarized in the box below.

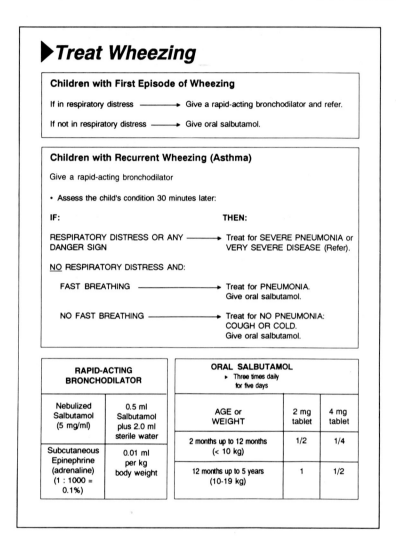

▶ Treat Wheezing

Children with First Episode of Wheezing

If in respiratory distress ⟶ Give a rapid-acting bronchodilator and refer.

If not in respiratory distress ⟶ Give oral salbutamol.

Children with Recurrent Wheezing (Asthma)

Give a rapid-acting bronchodilator

• Assess the child's condition 30 minutes later:

IF:	THEN:
RESPIRATORY DISTRESS OR ANY DANGER SIGN ⟶	Treat for SEVERE PNEUMONIA or VERY SEVERE DISEASE (Refer).

NO RESPIRATORY DISTRESS AND:

FAST BREATHING ⟶	Treat for PNEUMONIA. Give oral salbutamol.
NO FAST BREATHING ⟶	Treat for NO PNEUMONIA: COUGH OR COLD. Give oral salbutamol.

RAPID-ACTING BRONCHODILATOR	
Nebulized Salbutamol (5 mg/ml)	0.5 ml Salbutamol plus 2.0 ml sterile water
Subcutaneous Epinephrine (adrenaline) (1 : 1000 = 0.1%)	0.01 ml per kg body weight

ORAL SALBUTAMOL ▶ Three times daily for five days		
AGE or WEIGHT	2 mg tablet	4 mg tablet
2 months up to 12 months (< 10 kg)	1/2	1/4
12 months up to 5 years (10-19 kg)	1	1/2

Essential skills and knowledge

By the end of this chapter, you should be able to do the following:

• Give an antibiotic in tablet (or syrup) form to children or young infants, if indicated.

• Teach mothers how to continue treatment at home and to provide home care.

• Select the appropriate method of treating fever in a child aged 2 months up to 5 years.

• Treat a child with a first episode of wheezing and assess a child who has recurrent wheezing.

PART 2
Management of the child with an ear problem or sore throat

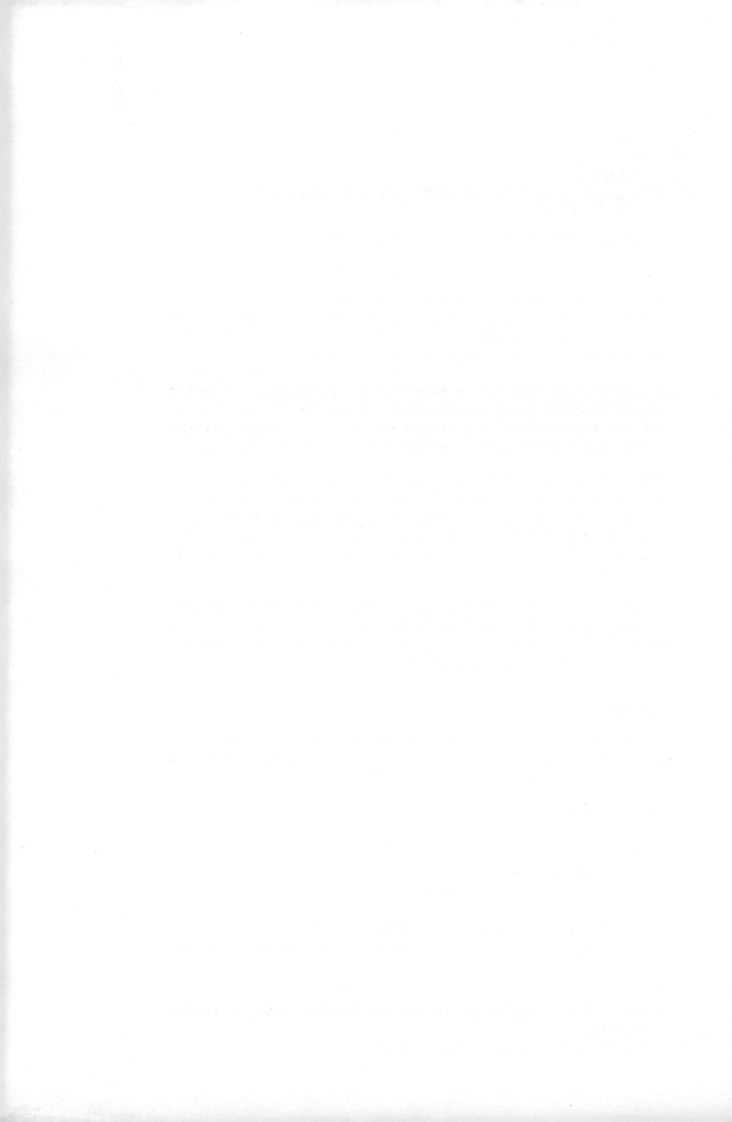

CHAPTER 6
Managing the child with an ear problem

The middle ear is considered a part of the respiratory tract. It is connected to the throat (pharynx) by the Eustachian tube. The middle ear often becomes infected when there is an infection of the nose or throat. Although some ear infections are caused by viruses, most are caused by bacteria, and can therefore be treated with antibiotics.

Ear infections rarely cause death, but they cause many days of sickness in children each year. Sometimes infections can spread from the ear to the bone behind the ear (mastoiditis) or to the brain (meningitis). Such infections are the main cause of preventable deafness in developing countries, and deafness can cause learning problems in school.

When a child has an ear infection, pus collects behind the eardrum. This causes pain and often fever. If the infection is not treated, the eardrum may burst. When this occurs, the pus discharges and the pain, fever and other symptoms (e.g. irritability) may disappear, but the child has difficulty hearing because the eardrum has a hole in it. Sometimes the eardrum heals by itself. However, at other times the discharge continues, the eardrum does not heal, and the child remains deaf in that ear.

As you read this section, refer to the fold-out chart, "Management of the Child with an Ear Problem or Sore Throat" at the back of this book. Look at the chart now and find the sections that describe how to manage a child with an ear problem. Locate the three steps: assess, classify the illness, and treatment instructions.

Assess

A mother may bring her child to the health centre because of ear pain or pus draining from the ear. If you have an otoscope and know how to use it, you should also look for an ear infection in any child who has an unexplained fever.

Assess the child by covering the points listed below.

Ask the mother (or caregiver) the following questions:

- **Does the child have ear pain?**
  If so, the child may have an ear infection.

- **Does the child have pus draining from the ear? For how long?**
  Pus draining from the ear is a sign of infection, even if the child no longer has pain.

Look or feel for the following:

- **Look for pus draining from the ear or a red, immobile eardrum (by pneumatic otoscopy).**
  Also, look to see if a foreign object is in the ear.

- **Feel for tender swelling behind the ear.**

  In young infants, the swelling may be *above* the ear.

The steps for assessing a child with an ear problem are summarized below and given on the left side of the fold-out chart under the title "Assess".

ASK:

- Does the child have ear pain?
- Does the child have pus draining from the ear? For how long?

LOOK, FEEL:

- Look for pus draining from the ear or red, immobile eardrum (by otoscopy).
- Feel for tender swelling behind ear.

Classify the illness

A child with an ear problem is classified as having either:

— mastoiditis,

— acute ear infection, or

— chronic ear infection.

Mastoiditis

A child who has *tender swelling behind the ear* (in infants, the swelling may be above the ear) is classified as having mastoiditis. Tender swelling behind the ear may indicate a deep infection in the mastoid bone.

Treatment

A child with mastoiditis needs treatment with antibiotics and may require surgery. Refer the child urgently to a hospital after giving the first dose of antibiotic. Give the same type and dose of antibiotic as for pneumonia (see Chapter 5).

Acute ear infection

A child who has *pus draining from the ear for less than 2 weeks, ear pain, or a red, immobile eardrum* (seen by pneumatic otoscopy) is classified as having an acute ear infection (acute otitis media). If you find a foreign object lodged in the ear, refer the child to a hospital for the object to be removed.

Treatment

The child should be given an antibiotic to treat the acute ear infection. Also dry the ear by wicking if pus is draining from the ear (see the next page for instructions on how to do this). Ear drops are not recommended because they keep the ear moist, and do not reach the infection.

Chronic ear infection

A child who has *pus draining from the ear for 2 weeks or more* is classified as having a chronic ear infection (chronic otitis media).

Treatment

The most important and effective treatment is to keep the ear dry by wicking (see below).

The bacteria that cause chronic ear infections are often different from those that cause acute ear infections. Thus, antibiotics are usually not effective against chronic ear infections, although a single course of an antibiotic is often tried in children with a chronic ear infection. (Follow the guidelines of your national ARI programme.) Antibiotic treatment should not replace drying the ear. Do not give repeated courses of antibiotics for a chronic ear infection.

Children who do *not* have tender swelling behind the ear, pus draining from the ear, ear pain, or a red, immobile eardrum are not put into any of the three classifications described above. Although these children might have an ear problem (e.g. an infected insect bite in the ear), it is not considered a respiratory problem and will not be discussed further.

Below is the section of the chart that summarizes the management of the child with an ear infection.

CLASSIFY THE ILLNESS

SIGNS:	• Tender swelling behind the ear.	• Pus draining from the ear LESS than two weeks, or • Ear pain, or • Red, immobile eardrum (by otoscopy).	• Pus draining from the ear two weeks or MORE.
CLASSIFY AS:	**MASTOIDITIS**	**ACUTE EAR INFECTION**	**CHRONIC EAR INFECTION**
TREATMENT:	▸ Refer URGENTLY to hospital. ▸ Give first dose of antibiotic. ▸ Treat fever, if present. ▸ Give paracetamol for pain.	▸ Give an antibiotic for five days, as for pneumonia. ▸ Dry the ear by wicking. ▸ Reassess in five days. ▸ Treat fever, if present. ▸ Give paracetamol for pain.	▸ Dry the ear by wicking. ▸ Treat fever, if present. ▸ Give paracetamol for pain.

Treatment instructions

Dry the ear by wicking

Dry the child's ear for the first time in the health centre. *Use this opportunity to demonstrate to the mother how she should dry the child's ear at home.*

1. Roll a clean, soft, absorbent, cotton cloth into a wick. Never use a cotton-tipped applicator or stick of any kind. Do not use paper (see Fig. 7a).
2. Place the wick in the child's ear (see Fig. 7b).
3. Remove the wick when it is wet.
4. Replace the wick with a clean one, and repeat these steps until the ear is dry.

The mother should dry the ear this way at least three times a day at home, until the ear stays dry. It usually takes 1–2 weeks for the ear to stop draining and stay dry. The mother often

(a)

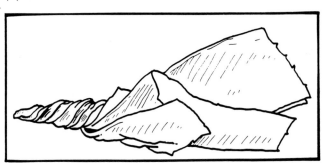

(b)

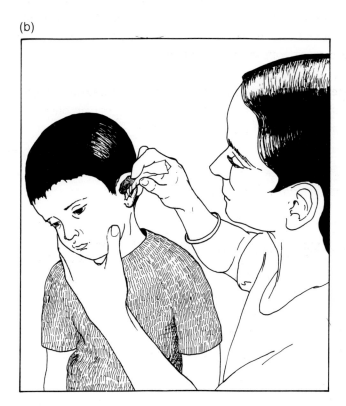

Fig. 7. **Drying the ear by wicking.**

needs assistance to learn how to dry the ear. Drying a draining ear is time-consuming for the mother but is the most effective therapy.[1] Explain to her that although wicking takes a long time, not wicking the ear could cause the child to go deaf.

Precautions for a child with a draining ear

Also instruct the mother in these precautions for a child with a draining ear:

- Do not leave anything in the ear, such as cotton wool, between wicking treatments.
- Do not put oil or any other fluid into the ear.
- Do not let the child go swimming or get water in the ear.

---

[1] Some programmes will want to teach staff to gently syringe a draining ear with a small amount of clean water, to help clear the pus. Instructions on how to do this are given in the document, *Acute respiratory infections in children: case management in small hospitals in developing countries—a manual for doctors and other senior health workers* (available on request from the national ARI programme in your country).

The steps to follow when drying an ear by wicking are summarized in the box below.

▶ Dry the Ear by Wicking

▶ **To dry the ear:**
- ▶ Roll clean, absorbent cloth into a wick.
- ▶ Place the wick in the child's ear.
- ▶ Remove the wick when wet.
- ▶ Replace the wick with a clean one until the ear is dry.

Give an antibiotic

Refer to the box, "Give an oral antibiotic for an ear infection", for information about antibiotic dosages (see below). The antibiotics listed in this box are also used to treat pneumonia. See Chapter 5 for instructions on how to give these antibiotics and how to instruct the mother to complete the antibiotic treatment at home.

If the child has an acute ear infection, ask the mother to bring the child back in 5 days. Repeat the same course of antibiotic if the child has not improved. For chronic ear infections, drying the ear is the most important part of management.

▶ Give an Oral Antibiotic for an Ear Infection

- ▶ Give first dose of antibiotic in clinic.
- ▶ Instruct mother on how to give the antibiotic for five days at home.

AGE or WEIGHT	COTRIMOXAZOLE (trimethoprim + sulphamethoxazole) ▶ Two times daily for 5 days.			AMOXYCILLIN ▶ Three times daily for 5 days.		AMPICILLIN ▶ Four times daily for 5 days.	
	Adult Tablet single strength (80 mg trimethoprim + 400 mg sulphamethoxazole)	Pediatric Tablet (20 mg trimethoprim + 100 mg sulphamethoxazole)	Syrup (40 mg trimethoprim + 200 mg sulphamethoxazole per 5 ml)	Tablet 250 mg	Syrup 125 mg in 5 ml	Tablet 250 mg	Syrup 250 mg in 5 ml
Less than 2 months (< 5 kg) *	1/4*	1*	2.5 ml*	1/4	2.5 ml	1/2	2.5 ml
2 months up to 12 months (6-9 kg)	1/2	2	5 ml	1/2	5 ml	1	5 ml
12 months up to 5 years (10-19 kg)	1	3	7.5 ml	1	10 ml	1	5 ml

    * Give oral antibiotic for 5 days at home only if referral is not feasible.

    * If the child is less than 1 month old, give 1/2 pediatric tablet or 1.25 ml syrup twice daily.
     Avoid cotrimoxazole in infants less than one month of age who are premature or jaundiced.

Give paracetamol

If the child has pain or a high fever (39°C or above), paracetamol can be given. See Chapter 5 for details on how to give paracetamol.

Essential skills and knowledge

By the end of this chapter, you should be able to assess, classify and appropriately treat the child with an ear problem.

CHAPTER 7
Managing the child with a sore throat

One of the most frequent symptoms of common cold is a sore throat. The majority of sore throats are due to viruses, and get better in a few days with good home care, and no additional treatment. Most children only need a safe, soothing remedy for a sore throat, to keep the throat moist.

However, some children with a sore throat require an antibiotic. Antibiotic treatment is necessary if the child develops a throat abscess or if a streptococcal throat infection is suspected. In particular, a child with a streptococcal sore throat (streptococcal pharyngitis, often called strep throat) needs to be treated with an effective antibiotic because the bacteria can cause rheumatic fever, a disease that involves the joints and weakens the heart. The purpose of antibiotic treatment is to kill all the streptococcal bacteria to prevent rheumatic fever.

As you read this section, refer to the fold-out chart, "Management of the Child with an Ear Problem or Sore Throat" at the back of this book. Look at the chart now and find the sections that describe how to manage a child with a sore throat. Locate the three steps of the management process: assess, classify the illness, and treatment instructions.

Assess

Assess the child with a sore throat by covering the points listed below.

Ask the mother the following question:

- **Is the child able to drink?**

Look and feel for the following:

- **Feel the front of the neck for nodes.**
  Feel the glands in the front of the neck to see if they are enlarged and tender. If so, then:

- **Look for exudate on the throat.**
  Look at the throat with a light. See if there is a white exudate (white patches) on the throat.[1]

The steps for assessing a child with a sore throat are summarized below and given on the right side of the fold-out chart, under the title "Assess".

---

[1] In countries where diphtheria cases still occur, it is important to consider this possibility in children with a grey exudate on their throat. Annex 2 contains a detailed description of management of vaccine-preventable acute respiratory infections, including diphtheria.

ASK: • Is the child able to drink?	***LOOK, FEEL:*** • Feel the front of the neck for nodes. • Look for exudate on the throat.

Classify the illness

Most children with a sore throat will get better in a few days with good home care, which includes giving a safe, soothing remedy to keep the throat moist. However, some children with a sore throat need antibiotic treatment. These children are classified as having either:

— throat abscess, or
— streptococcal sore throat.

Throat abscess

A child who is *not able to drink at all* is classified as having a throat abscess. Although it is not common, children may develop abscesses at the back of the throat or around the tonsils, which make it difficult for them to swallow.

Treatment

Refer the child to a hospital for treatment and, if needed, for the abscess to be drained. Give benzathine penicillin[1] by intramuscular injection.

Streptococcal sore throat (streptococcal pharyngitis)

A child who has *tender, enlarged lymph nodes in the front of the neck, and a white exudate on the throat* is classified as having streptococcal sore throat.

Treatment

Give a single injection of benzathine penicillin to prevent rheumatic fever from developing. Many mothers will not complete the required 10-day treatment with an oral antibiotic. Therefore, an injection of benzathine penicillin is preferred for suspected streptococcal sore throat. Co-trimoxazole[2] should *not* be given because it is not as effective.

Children who are able to drink, do not have tender, enlarged lymph nodes in the front of the neck, and do not have a white exudate on the throat, are not put into either of the two categories listed above. These children will get better in a few days with good home care, which includes giving a safe, soothing remedy to keep the throat moist.

Below is the section of the chart that summarizes the management of the child with a throat infection.

---

[1] INN = benzathine benzylpenicillin.
[2] INN = trimethoprim–sulfamethoxazole.

CLASSIFY THE ILLNESS

SIGNS:	• Not able to drink.	• Tender, enlarged lymph node on neck **and** • White exudate on throat.
CLASSIFY AS:	**THROAT ABSCESS**	**STREPTOCOCCAL SORE THROAT**
TREATMENT:	▶ Refer to hospital. ▶ Give benzathine penicillin. ▶ Treat fever, if present. ▶ Give paracetamol for pain.	▶ Give benzathine penicillin. ▶ Give safe, soothing remedy for sore throat. ▶ Treat fever, if present. ▶ Give paracetamol for pain.

Treatment instructions

- **Soothe the throat with a safe remedy.**

  Ask the mother to soothe the child's throat by giving the child warm, sweetened drinks to sip, such as tea and honey[1] (see page 41).

- **Give paracetamol.**

  Give paracetamol if the child is in pain or has a high fever. Refer to Chapter 5 for details of how to administer paracetamol.

- **Give an antibiotic.**

  Give an antibiotic to children who are classified as having streptococcal sore throat. Whenever possible, give benzathine penicillin by intramuscular injection. (Use the chart on the next page to determine the appropriate dosage.)

  If only oral antibiotics are available, give amoxycillin,[2] ampicillin or penicillin V[3,4] for 10 days. Refer to the box, "Give an oral antibiotic for an ear infection" to determine the appropriate dosage.

  Note that a child with streptococcal sore throat is given a longer-lasting antibiotic than the child with pneumonia. This does *not* mean that streptococcal sore throat is a more serious disease than pneumonia. A child with streptococcal sore throat receives long-lasting antibiotics because:

  - Treatment with a long-lasting antibiotic such as benzathine penicillin, or oral antibiotics for 10 days, is required to kill all the streptococcal bacteria. If you do not kill all the bacteria, there may be later complications (such as a weak heart from rheumatic fever).

  - Bacterial pneumonia can be cured with 5 days of antibiotic treatment.

---

[1] Some health centres will provide an effective, soothing remedy for sore throat. See the discussion of home care in Chapter 5.
[2] INN = amoxicillin.
[3] INN = phenoxymethylpenicillin.
[4] Co-trimoxazole is not recommended for streptococcal sore throat because it is not as effective. The recommended dose of penicillin V is 12.5 mg per kg of body weight every 6 hours, or 25 mg per kg of body weight every 12 hours, for 10 days.

Use the box below to determine the correct dosage of benzathine penicillin.

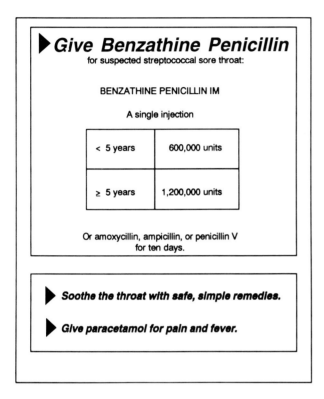

▶ *Give Benzathine Penicillin*
for suspected streptococcal sore throat:

BENZATHINE PENICILLIN IM

A single injection

< 5 years	600,000 units
≥ 5 years	1,200,000 units

Or amoxycillin, ampicillin, or penicillin V
for ten days.

▶ *Soothe the throat with safe, simple remedies.*

▶ *Give paracetamol for pain and fever.*

Essential skills and knowledge

By the end of this chapter, you should be able to assess, classify and appropriately treat the child with a sore throat.

ANNEX 1
Checklist of essential skills and knowledge

In order to manage acute respiratory infections, the health worker should be able to:

1. Select the appropriate case management chart for assessing, classifying and treating acute respiratory infections:

   • For a child with cough or difficult breathing, the health worker should use the chart, "Management of the Child with Cough or Difficult Breathing".

   • For a child with only an ear problem or sore throat, the health worker should use the chart, "Management of the Child with an Ear Problem or Sore Throat".

2. Assess a child (ask, look and listen) for danger signs of very severe disease and pneumonia, and check for other signs of the child's general condition.

3. Classify the illness of the child aged 2 months up to 5 years with cough and difficult breathing, based on signs found during the assessment.

Classification	Corresponding signs
Very severe disease	Not able to drink, convulsions, abnormally sleepy or difficult to wake, stridor when calm, or severe malnutrition
Severe pneumonia	Chest indrawing
Pneumonia	No chest indrawing, and fast breathing
No pneumonia: cough or cold	No chest indrawing, and no fast breathing

4. Select appropriate treatment for the child aged 2 months up to 5 years, based on the above classifications: refer, give an antibiotic, or advise the mother to give home care.

5. Classify the illness of a young infant (aged less than 2 months) with cough or difficult breathing, based on signs found during the assessment.

Classification	Corresponding signs
Very severe disease	Stopped feeding well, convulsions, abnormally sleepy or difficult to wake, stridor when calm, wheezing, fever or low body temperature
Severe pneumonia	Fast breathing (60 times per minute or more), or severe chest indrawing
No pneumonia: cough or cold	No fast breathing (less than 60 times per minute) and no severe chest indrawing or danger signs

6. Select appropriate treatment for the young infant, based on the above classifications: refer, or advise the mother to give home care.

7. Give an antibiotic in tablet (or syrup) form or by injection to children or young infants, if indicated.

8. Teach mothers how to continue antibiotic treatment at home and provide home care.

9. Select the appropriate method of treating fever in a child aged 2 months up to 5 years.

10. Treat a child with a first episode of wheezing and assess a child who has recurrent wheezing.

11. Assess, classify and appropriately treat a child with an ear problem.

12. Assess, classify and appropriately treat a child with a sore throat.

I.

ANNEX 2
Managing vaccine-preventable acute respiratory infections: measles, pertussis and diphtheria

Acute respiratory infections that can be prevented by immunization, such as measles, pertussis and diphtheria, still occur in most countries. If these infections are not treated promptly, they can cause deaths in children. Therefore, it is important that health workers recognize these diseases and provide the correct treatment.

Measles

Measles and pneumonia

Pneumonia is a common cause of death from measles. Pneumonia can be caused by the measles virus itself or by a bacterial infection. The case management guidelines for acute respiratory infections summarized in this manual are also applicable to pneumonia complicating measles.

Recognizing measles

A child with measles has fever, a generalized rash and a cough, a runny nose or red eyes. The fever is usually present for 3–4 days before the rash appears and the child may appear to have a common cold with a cough, a runny nose or red eyes. The rash is red and begins behind the ears and on the forehead, and then spreads to the rest of the body. There are no blisters or pustules. The rash fades after 5–6 days and may leave brown marks on the skin. The skin also often peels.

Assessing, classifying and treating acute respiratory infections in a child aged 2 months up to 5 years with measles

Children aged 2 months up to 5 years with measles and a cough or difficult breathing should be assessed as described in Chapter 3: look for danger signs, count the breathing rate, look for chest indrawing and listen for stridor. Children with danger signs, including stridor when calm, or chest indrawing should be given a first dose of antibiotics and vitamin A and then referred urgently to hospital.

If a child has fast breathing without danger signs or chest indrawing, the child should be treated with antibiotics and vitamin A at home. Ask the mother to return with the child in 2 days (or earlier if the child is getting worse). If the child has not improved within 2 days, refer the child to hospital (see Annex 3). You should also carry out the following assessment:

1. Ask the mother if the child has ear pain or pus draining from the ear. If so, the child may have an ear infection (see Chapter 6). Acute ear infection is a common complication of measles.

60

2. Check the child's eyes for corneal clouding (loss of visual clarity) and for pus draining from the eyes. If the child has corneal clouding, he or she should be treated with tetracycline eye ointment and given a dose of vitamin A and then referred urgently to hospital. Measles can cause corneal ulceration and blindness. Conjunctivitis, an inflammation of the white part of the eye, is a common complication of measles and should be treated with tetracycline eye ointment; the mother should be advised to bring the child back after 2 days if pus is still draining from the child's eyes.

3. Check the child's mouth for signs of redness or soreness and for mouth ulcers. Stomatitis, an inflammation of the inside of the mouth, can complicate measles and contribute to malnutrition by making feeding difficult. If the child has deep or extensive mouth ulcers, refer the child to hospital. If the child's mouth is red or sore, apply gentian violet to the affected part. Show the mother how to feed the child with a cup and spoon if the child is unable to breast-feed. Advise the mother to return with the child if he or she is unable to feed or is losing weight.

If the child has diarrhoea, assess, classify and treat the child using the chart *Management of the Patient with Diarrhoea.*[1]

Tell the mother to have her other children immunized against measles immediately, if they are not already immunized.

To prevent weight loss, children with measles should be given energy-rich and nutrient-rich foods (see page 40) and encouraged to eat frequently.

Vitamin A treatment

Children with measles and an acute respiratory infection should be given two doses of vitamin A. Show the mother how to administer the vitamin A and watch while she gives the first dose in the clinic. Then give her a second capsule to administer at home the next day. The dose is as follows:

Age	Recommended dose of vitamin A		
	Capsules, 200 000 IU	Capsules, 100 000 IU	Oily solution, 100 000 IU/ml in multidose dispenser
Up to 6 months	—	1/2 capsule	0.5 ml
6–12 months	1/2 capsule	1 capsule	1.0 ml
12 months up to 5 years	1 capsule	2 capsules	2.0 ml

Children who have had measles remain at high risk

Children who have had measles may be at high risk of serious infections for several months

---

[1] Available on request from the Division of Diarrhoeal and Acute Respiratory Disease Control, World Health Organization, 1211 Geneva 27, Switzerland.

after the illness. Advise the mother to return with the child if he or she develops a cough or difficult breathing, is not able to drink, passes blood in the stool or is very sick. If possible, arrange to see the child after 2 weeks to reassess the child.

Pertussis (whooping cough)

Recognizing pertussis

The first signs of pertussis are a cough and a cold. After 7–10 days, the cough becomes distressing and spasmodic. During an episode of pertussis, a child may cough violently 10–30 times before he or she can finally pull air back into the lungs with a noisy "whoop" when breathing in. The cough often causes vomiting. The child may also turn blue or have convulsions. Between bouts of coughing, the child may look well. In infants, however, the main sign of pertussis may be long periods of not breathing (apnoea).

An attack of pertussis may last for weeks or even months. This places a great strain on the child and the family and interferes with nutrition.

Treatment

Children with pertussis should be referred to hospital if:

- they are less than 6 months of age;
- they have complications such as convulsions or periods of apnoea, or turn blue after coughing;
- they have severe pneumonia, severe dehydration or severe malnutrition.

A child with pertussis may vomit frequently and become malnourished. To prevent weight loss, teach the mother to give the child energy-rich and nutrient-rich foods and to offer food frequently. Advise the mother that pertussis often lasts for 6–8 weeks. Ask her to return with the child if the child is not able to eat and is losing weight, begins to breathe fast or has a convulsion, or turns blue after coughing.

Pertussis and pneumonia

Pneumonia is the most common complication and the most frequent cause of death in pertussis, especially in infants. It should be treated with antibiotics, as described in Chapter 5.

Diphtheria

In countries where diphtheria still occurs, it is important to consider the possibility of this disease in children with an acute respiratory infection who present with stridor or an exudate on the throat.

Recognizing diphtheria

Diphtheria is characterized by the formation of a greyish membrane that adheres to the throat and cannot be removed with a swab. Be very gentle when examining the child's throat, because it is possible to obstruct the airway with the membrane. If you are not sure whether the child has diphtheria, refer the child to hospital.

Treatment

Children suspected of having diphtheria need to be referred urgently to hospital for treatment with penicillin and diphtheria antitoxin. They should receive a first dose of antibiotics, preferably a penicillin, before referral.

ANNEX 3
Referring a child to a hospital

Rationale for referral

A referral should only be made if you expect the child will receive better care at another facility. In some cases, giving the child the best care you have available is better than sending the child on a long trip to a referral hospital that may not have the supplies, equipment or expertise to care for the child.

Referring the child

The following are recommended steps in referring a child to a hospital:

1. Explain to the mother that her child needs treatment in a hospital. Get her agreement to take the child. If she says that she does not want to take the child, identify her reasons. Help calm her fears and solve other difficulties she may have.

2. Discuss with the mother how she can travel to the hospital.

3. Give the child the first dose of an antibiotic, if indicated. Do not delay referral if this medicine cannot be given promptly.

   - If you only have an oral antibiotic, give the antibiotic only if the child is able to drink and can swallow the antibiotic safely.

   - If there is a long referral time, provide the mother with additional doses of the antibiotic to give the child during the trip (at the appropriate dosing schedule).

   - If the mother seems unwilling to take the child, give her the full 5-day course of the antibiotic.

4. Ensure that the mother keeps the young infant warm during the journey. Small and sick infants lose heat rapidly, especially when they are wet. Feel the young infant's hands and feet. They should be warm. Keeping the young infant warm is especially important.

   To maintain the body temperature, keep the young infant dry and well wrapped. A hat or bonnet will help to prevent heat loss from the head. Ask the mother to keep her young infant next to her body, ideally between her breasts. Also keep the room warm, if possible.

5. Give any other treatment that may be needed, such as in the case of fever, wheezing or suspected cerebral malaria.

6. Write a referral note for the mother to take with her to the hospital. Tell her to give it to the health worker who sees her child. Include the following information:

- The signs you have seen.
- How you classified the illness.
- The treatment that you have given.
- Any other information that the health worker at the referral facility needs to know in order to care for the child, such as earlier treatment of the illness.

ANNEX 4
When referral is not feasible

The best treatment for a child with a very serious illness is at a hospital, if the hospital is able to provide adequate assessment and treatment.

However, referral is not always feasible. The hospital might be too far away, it may not have the equipment or expertise to care for the child, or adequate transportation might not be available. Occasionally parents refuse to take a child to a hospital, in spite of the efforts of the health worker to explain the need for referral.

If referral is not feasible, then the health worker should do whatever he or she can to help the family care for the child. This may mean arranging for the child to stay near the health centre so that you can see the child several times a day, or arranging for visits at home. Health workers can provide the following essential care.

1. Treat the child with an antibiotic (if indicated by the treatment plan).

The child aged 2 months up to 5 years
Intramuscular chloramphenicol is the best choice of a single antibiotic for a child with a severe infection. It is effective both for children who have severe pneumonia and for those with danger signs who may have meningitis, and can be given to children who are not able to drink. Give it for 5 days as specified in Table 1. Treat the child for at least 5 days. Continue the treatment for 3 days after the child is well.

Table 1 **Recommended antibiotic treatment for a child aged 2 months up to 5 years, when referral is not feasible**

Antibiotic	Recommended dose	Estimated single dose (in ml or capsules), according to body weight in kg				
		3–5 kg	6–9 kg	10–14 kg	15–19 kg	20–29 kg
Chloramphenicol powder for injection, 1 g (as sodium succinate) in vial, mixed with 4 ml of sterile water	25 mg/kg every 6 hours (maximum 1 g) for at least 5 days	0.5	1	1.5	2	2.5
	50 mg/kg every 12 hours (maximum 1 g) for at least 5 days	1	2	3	4	5
Oral suspension, 125 mg (as palmitate salt)/5 ml	25 mg/kg every 6 hours (maximum 1 g) for at least 5 days	6	8	12	15	–
Capsule, 250 mg	25 mg/kg every 6 hours (maximum 1 g) for at least 5 days	–	–	1	1	2

If parenteral chloramphenicol is not available, then the next best option is to give oral chloramphenicol by mouth or by nasogastric tube. The dosage is the same as for parenteral chloramphenicol.

If chloramphenicol is not available in any form, then give the child benzylpenicillin by intramuscular injection, or the oral antibiotic for pneumonia that you are using in your health centre by mouth or by nasogastric tube. Give the oral antibiotic for 5 days as specified in the box, "Give an antibiotic", on the fold-out chart "Management of the Child with Cough or Difficult Breathing". If the child vomits, repeat the dose.

The young infant

Give intramuscular benzylpenicillin and gentamicin for 5 days as specified in Table 2. Treat the young infant for at least 5 days. Continue the treatment for 3 days after the young infant is well.

If intramuscular benzylpenicillin and gentamicin are not available, then give the young infant the oral antibiotic for pneumonia that you are using in your health centre by mouth or by nasogastric tube. Give it for 5 days as specified in the box, "Give an antibiotic", on the fold-out chart. If the young infant vomits, repeat the dose.

2. Keep the young infant warm.
   Small and ill infants lose heat rapidly, especially when wet. Feel the young infant's hands and feet. They should be warm. Keeping the young infant warm is especially important.

To maintain the body temperature, keep the young infant dry and well wrapped. A hat or bonnet will help prevent heat loss from the head. Ask the mother to keep her young infant next to her body, ideally between her breasts. Also keep the room warm, if possible.

Table 2 **Recommended antibiotic treatment for a young infant aged less than 2 months, when referral is not feasible**

Antibiotic	Recommended dose, according to age		Estimated single dose (in ml), for 3–5-kg young infant
	First week of life	**Aged 1 week up to 2 months**	
Gentamicin[a]			
Injection, 10 mg/ml in 2-ml vial, undiluted	2.5 mg/kg every 12 hours for at least 5 days	2.5 mg/kg every 8 hours for at least 5 days	1
Injection, 40 mg/ml in 2-ml vial, diluted with 6 ml of sterile water	2.5 mg/kg every 12 hours for at least 5 days	2.5 mg/kg every 8 hours for at least 5 days	1
plus			
Benzylpenicillin[b]			
Powder for injection, 600 mg (= 1 million IU) in vial, diluted with 2 ml of sterile water	50 000 units/kg every 12 hours for at least 5 days	50 000 units/kg every 6 hours for at least 5 days	0.5

[a] When gentamicin is administered, it is preferable to calculate the exact dose based on the infant's weight and to avoid using 40 mg/ml gentamicin, undiluted.
[b] Also known as penicillin G.

3. Clear secretions.

   A blocked nose can interfere with feeding. If the infant's nose is blocked, use a plastic syringe to gently suck any secretions from the nose. (See Chapter 5 for instructions on clearing the nose.)

4. Treat fever, if present.

   Fever increases consumption of oxygen. In the child aged 2 months up to 5 years, control the fever by giving paracetamol every 6 hours. In areas where there is falciparum malaria, also give an antimalarial according to the guidelines of the national malaria programme in your country.

5. Manage the child's fluids carefully.

   Children with pneumonia or very severe disease can become overloaded with fluids easily. They should not be given too much fluid.

   On the other hand, children with pneumonia or very severe disease often lose fluids during a respiratory infection, especially if they also have a fever. They can go into shock if they do not receive adequate fluid. Therefore, you should give fluids cautiously.

   • Encourage the mother to continue breast-feeding, if the child is not in respiratory distress. If the child is too ill to breast-feed, the mother can express milk into a cup and feed the child with a spoon, slowly.

   • If the child is not able to drink and you know how to insert a nasogastric tube, do so. Avoid using a nasogastric tube if the child is in respiratory distress. Give milk or formula by nasogastric tube as follows until the child can drink:

     − aged less than 12 months: 5 ml/kg per hour.[1]
     − aged 12 months up to 5 years: 3–4 ml/kg per hour.[1]

   Alternatively, give the child frequent breast-feeds.

   • Avoid giving fluids intravenously, *unless* the child is in shock.

For more detailed information on dosage and duration of treatment, see the document *Acute respiratory infections in children: case management in small hospitals in developing countries. A manual for doctors and other senior health workers.*[2] Although the document is not written for health centres, it describes how to treat children with severe pneumonia and very severe disease, and might be useful in a health centre when there is no hospital for referral.

---

[1] The total in 24 hours:
− aged less than 12 months: 120 ml/kg;
− aged 12 months up to 5 years: 72–96 ml/kg.
[2] Available from the national ARI programme in your country.

ANNEX 5
Using a rapid-acting bronchodilator

Bronchodilators act rapidly when given by injection or inhaled as a vapour. This is why they are called "rapid-acting" bronchodilators. They can be used in a health centre to treat a child who is wheezing and in respiratory distress.

Salbutamol and epinephrine are two of the most common and effective bronchodilators. They should be administered as follows:

- Give epinephrine by subcutaneous injection.

- Give salbutamol by:

  - metered-dose inhaler. This is a small, hand-held canister of pressurized salbutamol with a spray valve, through which the child breathes in the vapour.
  - nebulizer. This is a device consisting of a container for a liquid mixture of salbutamol and water. The mixture can be vaporized using an electric air compressor or a continuous flow of oxygen at 6–8 litres per minute from a cylinder. An aerosol mask is attached to the top of the nebulizer to cover the nose and mouth, through which the child inhales the vapour. Alternatively, a footpump may be used to vaporize the salbutamol mixture. To be suitable for this purpose, the footpump must be robust, durable and easy to operate and maintain. It must also be free from oil and grease, which could contaminate the mixture and be inhaled by the child.

Giving epinephrine (adrenaline) by subcutaneous injection

Epinephrine (adrenaline) must be administered in very small doses. Epinephrine is available in two dilutions: 1:1000 and 1:10 000. Use the 1:1000 dilution; this contains 1 mg in 1 ml (a 0.1% solution).

To determine the dose, multiply the weight of the child in kilograms by 0.01 ml. For example, a child weighing 9 kg would receive 0.09 ml. Prepare the injection using a 1-ml syringe as shown in the figure below. If you are not certain about the size of syringe to use, look at a tuberculin syringe.

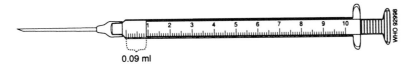

0.09 ml

This is a 1.0-ml syringe containing 0.09 ml of epinephrine

Giving salbutamol by metered-dose inhaler[1]

Children under 5 years old lack the coordination for using a metered-dose inhaler by themselves. They often cannot use the mouthpiece or breathe in when the inhaler is pressed. To overcome these problems, use a spacer device. This allows the salbutamol to be squirted into an enclosed space and the child inhales the vapour through a mask which is placed over the nose and mouth.

Spacer devices are available commercially, or can be made by modifying locally available containers, such as 1-litre plastic bottles or a plastic cup (see below).

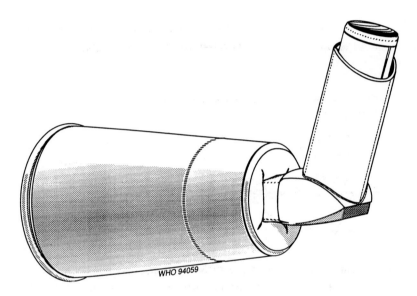

WHO 94059

A metered-dose inhaler attached to a plastic cup (volume 150 ml)

---

[1] For further instructions on the use of nebulizers, see *Bronchodilators and other medications for the treatment of wheeze-associated illnesses in young infants*. Geneva, World Health Organization, 1993 (unpublished document WHO/ARI/93.29; available on request from the Division of Diarrhoeal and Acute Respiratory Disease Control, World Health Organization, 1211 Geneva 27, Switzerland).

Glossary of terms used in this book

Acute: having a short course.

Acute cough: a cough lasting less than 30 days.

Acute ear infection: an ear infection lasting less than 14 days.

Acute respiratory infection: an acute infection of the ear, nose, throat, epiglottis, larynx, trachea, bronchi, bronchioles or lung.

    Acute lower respiratory infection (ALRI): an acute infection of the epiglottis, larynx, trachea, bronchi, bronchioles or lung.

    Acute upper respiratory infection (AURI): an acute infection of the nose, pharynx (throat) or middle ear.

Antibiotic: a drug that kills bacteria or inhibits their growth. Antibiotics are not effective against viruses. (Also referred to as an antimicrobial.)

Antimalarial: a drug that kills malaria parasites.

Apnoea: abnormally long periods of not breathing.

Asthma: a condition marked by repeated attacks of wheezing in which the airways narrow due to bronchospasm (see below), oedema of the mucosa, and mucus in the lumen of the bronchi and bronchioles (see below). (Also called wheezy bronchitis, although this term should be avoided.)

Bacteria: a kind of microorganism that is killed by antibiotics.

Breathing rate: number of breaths per minute. (Also referred to as respiratory rate.)

Bronchi: the large air passages of the lungs.

Bronchioles: the smallest air passages of the lungs.

Bronchiolitis: a viral infection of the bronchioles, which causes swelling and narrowing of the airways, resulting in wheezing. It can kill infants because of hypoxia or because pneumonia develops.

Bronchitis: inflammation of the bronchi, generally caused by a virus infection in young children.

Bronchodilator: a drug that helps to open the air passages of the lungs to relieve wheezing caused by contraction of the muscles around the airways.

Bronchospasm: spasmodic tightening or contraction of the muscles around the bronchi and bronchioles which narrows the airways and causes wheezing.

Chest indrawing: retraction or drawing in of the lower part of the chest (lower ribs and lower sternum) when a child breathes in. It is a sign of severe pneumonia, wheezing or croup. (Also called subcostal indrawing or subcostal retraction.)

Chronic: persisting for a long time.

Chronic cough: a cough lasting for at least 30 days.

Chronic ear infection: an ear infection lasting for at least 14 days. A child who has pus draining from the ear for 2 weeks or more is classified as having a chronic ear infection. (Also called chronic otitis media.)

Cold: an acute viral infection of the upper respiratory tract. (Also called common cold.)

Complication: a secondary disease or condition occurring during the course of a primary disease. For example, pneumonia may be a complication of measles.

Conjunctivitis: inflammation of the conjunctiva, the white part of the eye.

Convulsion: a violent uncontrolled contraction or series of contractions of the muscles, accompanied by a sudden loss of consciousness. Convulsions can be caused by high fever, meningitis, hypoxia, cerebral malaria, epilepsy or other conditions. (Also called fits.)

Croup: a condition resulting from narrowing of the larynx, trachea or epiglottis, which interferes with air entering the lungs. It can be caused by a viral or bacterial infection.

Cyanosis: a bluish, purplish coloration of the skin due to hypoxia.

Dehydration: the condition that results from loss of a large amount of water and salt from the body.

Diphtheria: an acute, contagious bacterial infection characterized by the formation of a grey, adherent membrane on the throat, nose or larynx. It may cause death from obstruction of the larynx or from cardiovascular complications resulting from the effects of toxin released from the site of infection. It is a vaccine-preventable disease.

Epiglottis: the lid-like cartilaginous structure overhanging the entrance to the larynx and serving to prevent food from entering the larynx and trachea during swallowing.

Epiglottitis: a bacterial infection of the epiglottis, which causes severe croup.

Epinephrine: a bronchodilator. It is given by subcutaneous injection. (Also called adrenaline.)

Eustachian tube: the tube that connects the throat to the middle ear. (Also called auditory tube.)

External auditory canal: the passage of the external ear leading to the eardrum.

Exudate: fluid, such as pus or discharge, formed as a result of injury or infection. It appears as white patches on the throat in streptococcal sore throat, and as a greyish membrane on the throat in diphtheria.

Fast breathing: 40 breaths per minute or more if the child is aged 12 months up to 5 years; 50 breaths per minute or more if the child is aged 2 months up to 12 months; 60 breaths per minute or more if the child is aged less than 2 months.

Feedback: information provided by others on the way a person is doing something. For example, managers are giving feedback when they inform their staff of work they are doing well or make suggestions for improvements.

Fit: see Convulsion.

Foreign body: an object that is not normal to the place where it is found. For example, a bean that is found in a child's airway.

Grunting: deep, short sounds that a child makes when he or she has difficulty breathing out. It is a sign of severe pneumonia.

Hypothermia: a low body temperature (less than 35.5 °C).

Hypoxia: not having enough oxygen in the body.

Jaundice: a sign of disease in which parts of the body, such as the eyes, turn yellow.

Kwashiorkor: a form of severe malnutrition caused by a lack of protein in the diet. A child with kwashiorkor may have an enlarged liver, a generalized swelling of the body (oedema), flaking, dry skin and thin, weak hair.

Laryngitis: an infection of the larynx which causes hoarseness or croup.

Laryngotracheitis: an infection of the larynx and trachea.

Larynx: a part of the airway which is between the epiglottis and trachea. (Also called the voice box.)

Marasmus: the most common form of severe malnutrition, which is characterized by severe muscle wasting and a lack of subcutaneous fat, giving the child a "skin and bones" appearance.

Mastoiditis: an infection of the mastoid bone (behind the ear.)

Measles: an acute infectious viral disease marked by fever, red spots on the skin, and conjunctivitis. It can cause stomatitis, which interferes with feeding. Pneumonia and diarrhoea are common complications. Measles is a vaccine-preventable disease.

Metered-dose inhaler: a small, hand-held device used for giving nebulized salbutamol.

Middle ear: the space behind the eardrum. It is connected to the throat by the Eustachian tube.

Nasal flaring: widening of the nose as the child breathes in. It is a sign of severe pneumonia.

Nebulizer: a device for pressurizing a liquid into vapour or spray. It is used for giving salbutamol.

Otitis media: an infection of the middle ear.

Otoscope: a device for examining the eardrum.

Paracetamol: a drug which lowers fever and relieves pain. (Also known as acetaminophen.)

Parenteral: not taken orally but rather by injection through some other route, e.g. under the skin (subcutaneous), into a vein (intravenous), or into a muscle (intramuscular).

Pertussis: an infectious bacterial disease, characterized by a series of short coughs, followed by a noise called a whoop when the child breathes in. The cough often causes vomiting. Pertussis is a vaccine-preventable disease. (Also known as whooping cough.)

Pharyngitis: an infection of the throat.

Pharynx: the throat.

Pneumatic otoscope: an otoscope equipped with a device to inject air into, and withdraw it from, the external auditory canal. It is used to diagnose otitis media, which is characterized by a reduction in or loss of movement of the eardrum.

Pneumonia: an acute infection of the lungs. It is classified according to severity based on clinical signs.

In the child aged 2 months up to 5 years:

Pneumonia: Cough or difficult breathing with fast breathing **but no** chest indrawing.

Severe pneumonia: cough or difficult breathing with chest indrawing.

In the young infant aged less than 2 months:

Severe pneumonia: severe chest indrawing or fast breathing. (Since pneumonia in a young infant can progress very rapidly to death, all pneumonia is considered severe in this age group.)

Respiratory distress: discomfort from not getting enough air into the lungs.

Respiratory rate: see Breathing rate.

Salbutamol: a bronchodilator. Available in tablet, syrup or liquid form. Liquid salbutamol is delivered by a nebulizer or by a metered-dose inhaler.

Sepsis: a condition caused by the presence of bacteria or their toxins in the blood. (Also called septicaemia or blood-poisoning.)

Sterile: free from living microorganisms, including viruses and bacteria.

Stomatitis: inflammation of the mouth.

Streptococcal sore throat: a throat infection caused by streptococcal bacteria. It is characterized by tender, enlarged lymph nodes in the front of the neck, and a white exudate on the throat. (Also called septic sore throat.)

Stridor: a harsh sound that a child makes when breathing in. It occurs when there is a narrowing of the larynx, trachea or epiglottis. Stridor can be caused by croup or a foreign body.

Throat abscess: an infection of the throat, resulting in the accumulation of pus.

Timer: a simple device allowing the accurate measurement of a time interval.

Trachea: the tube that connects the larynx to the bronchi. (Also called the windpipe.)

Tuberculosis: a chronic infectious disease caused by mycobacteria, characterized by a chronic cough and sometimes fever, weight loss and infection of lymph nodes. (Also known as TB.)

Virus: a microscopic infectious agent that cannot be killed by antibiotics.

Wheeze: a soft whistling noise that a child makes when breathing out. It may be caused by swelling and narrowing of the small airways of the lung or by contraction of the smooth muscles surrounding the airways in the lung.

Whooping cough: see Pertussis.

Wick: a strip of rolled, absorbent cotton cloth which is used to dry an ear that is draining.

Young infant: For the purposes of this book, a young infant is defined as a child less than 2 months old (0–1 month).

Fold-out charts